Ultrasound-guided Musculoskeletal Embolotherapies using the "Dochu" Technique

Yuji Okuno • Ralph Rogers
Alexander Loizides

Ultrasound-guided Musculoskeletal Embolotherapies using the "Dochu" Technique

Springer

Yuji Okuno
Musculoskeletal Intervention Center
Okuno Clinic
Tokyo, Japan

Alexander Loizides
Department of Radiology
Medical University Innsbruck
Innsbruck, Tirol, Austria

Ralph Rogers
Rogers Regenerative Medical Group
London, UK

ISBN 978-3-032-17249-5 ISBN 978-3-032-17250-1 (eBook)
https://doi.org/10.1007/978-3-032-17250-1

This Springer imprint is published by the registered company Springer Nature Switzerland AG
The registered company address is: Gewerbestrasse 11, 6330 Cham, Switzerland

Preface

The Purpose of This Book: For Whom and Why?

This textbook is written with a singular aim: to bring the Dochu technique into *real-world clinical practice.*

Through detailed photographs, ultrasound images, procedural steps, and anatomical guidance, the book is designed to serve as a *practical manual* for clinicians—particularly those outside the field of interventional radiology—who wish to incorporate Dochu into their practice.

Each chapter focuses on a specific disease or anatomical region, offering step-by-step instruction and case-based learning to guide implementation and build procedural confidence.

This book is not a theoretical treatise. It is the culmination of over a decade of hands-on development and clinical refinement. It is for the *general practitioner seeking new solutions*, the *specialist searching for less invasive options*, and the *sports physician looking to extend athletes careers.*

By simplifying embolization without compromising safety or science, we hope to make this promising therapy *available to more people, in more places, with greater impact.*

Tokyo, Japan — Yuji Okuno
London, UK — Ralph Rogers
Innsbruck, Tirol, Austria — Alexander Loizides

Contents

1 Introduction

Rethinking Embolization—From Radical Idea to Clinical Reality

> Embolizing the arteries around a joint to relieve pain? That sounds reckless—dangerous, even foolish.

Such is the natural reaction from anyone encountering this idea for the first time. It defies our basic understanding of vascular physiology and joint health. Isn't blood flow necessary for healing and preservation? Doesn't embolization mean necrosis, nerve damage, and joint destruction?

This skepticism is not only understandable—it is logical. For decades, interventional procedures involving embolization have been associated with stopping life-threatening hemorrhages, treating tumors, or managing acute vascular anomalies. The thought of deliberately occluding arteries supplying joints, muscles, tendons, or ligaments—structures essential for mobility and everyday function—seems counterintuitive at best, catastrophic at worst.

And yet, over the past decade, this idea has transformed from controversial hypothesis to clinical practice, under the framework of *transcatheter arterial microembolization (TAME)*. No longer confined to theoretical discussions, TAME is now performed across multiple countries and institutions, demonstrating both safety and efficacy in treating chronic musculoskeletal pain conditions. Clinical data from Europe, Asia, and North America increasingly support its utility in conditions such as osteoarthritis, adhesive capsulitis (frozen shoulder), epicondylitis, and chronic tendinopathies.

In fact, multiple peer-reviewed studies have shown significant reductions in pain scores, improvement in function, and sustained benefit for many patients who previously had limited options. For example, clinical trials have shown improvements of 50% or more in Visual Analog Scale (VAS) pain scores following genicular artery embolization for knee osteoarthritis. Furthermore, these procedures are associated with low complication rates and minimal recovery times, making them attractive alternatives to systemic pharmacotherapy or invasive surgery.

Y. Okuno et al., *Ultrasound-guided Musculoskeletal Embolotherapies using the "Dochu" Technique*, https://doi.org/10.1007/978-3-032-17250-1_1

So, how is such a seemingly dangerous concept possible?

The key lies in the nature of the embolic material used. Unlike traditional embolization, which often employs permanent particles or coils, *TAME utilizes temporary embolic agents* that dissolve within minutes to hours. A commonly used example is imipenem/cilastatin (IPM/CS), which acts transiently in the vasculature. In normal arteries, where endothelial integrity and flow dynamics are preserved, recanalization occurs rapidly, and tissue perfusion is restored before any meaningful ischemia can develop. However, in *abnormal neovasculature*, especially the immature, fragile vessels associated with chronic inflammation, the flow is sluggish and the vessels are prone to collapse. In these pathological contexts, even short-lived embolization is sufficient to cause vessel regression and symptom improvement.

But don't all blood vessels play a beneficial role?

That assumption, too, has been challenged by modern vascular biology. Since the early 2000s, researchers have distinguished between physiological angiogenesis (as seen in wound healing or development) and *pathological angiogenesis*, which occurs in chronic inflammatory environments. In diseases such as rheumatoid arthritis, chronic tendinopathies, and osteoarthritis, aberrant neovascularization is now recognized as a *driver of inflammation* and pain, rather than a compensatory or healing process. These abnormal vessels not only supply inflammatory mediators, but they also provide conduits for sensory nerve in growth—specifically, nociceptive C-fibers—into tissues where they do not belong, such as cartilage or tendon insertions. The result is a vicious cycle of pain, inflammation, and tissue degradation.

In this light, the concept of targeting and reducing pathological neovessels is not only plausible—it is scientifically sound.

Chronic Pain: An Unsolved Frontier

Chronic musculoskeletal pain remains one of the most burdensome medical challenges of our time. Nonsteroidal anti-inflammatory drugs (NSAIDs), corticosteroid injections, physical therapy, and surgery each offer benefits, but also limitations. Long-term drug use carries systemic risks, surgeries involve downtime and complications, and many patients remain undertreated—living with persistent pain that erodes quality of life.

In this context, *embolization provides a new therapeutic option*, particularly for patients who fall into the "treatment gap": those who are not candidates for surgery, or who have failed conservative therapies but are reluctant to pursue more aggressive interventions. By addressing the vascular and neurogenic contributors to pain, embolization offers a mechanism-based approach that complements, rather than competes with, existing modalities.

Democratizing Embolization: The Birth of "Dochu"

Traditionally, embolization has been the domain of highly trained interventional radiologists, performed in specialized angiography suites equipped with fluoroscopy, radiation shielding, and catheterization tools. The skill and equipment required have restricted access to a small number of physicians in large centers, effectively excluding most primary care physicians, sports physicians, orthopedic surgeons, rheumatologists, and outpatient providers from utilizing this therapy.

But what if embolization could be *simplified*?

What if it could be performed in a standard outpatient clinic, within minutes, *without fluoroscopy, catheters, or radiation*?

This book introduces such a method—*a simplified approach to embolization we refer to as "Dochu"* (short for Doumyaku-Chuusha, or "arterial injection" in Japanese). Developed through years of clinical refinement, Dochu allows physicians to identify and treat target arteries using *ultrasound-guided direct injection techniques*, applying temporary embolic agents directly to the inflamed vasculature. It is a practical, low-risk procedure that can be performed during a standard office visit, expanding access to embolization to a much broader group of practitioners and patients.

Diseases such as Heberden's nodes, rheumatoid arthritis, knee osteoarthritis, and even some post-traumatic conditions can now be approached using this minimally invasive method. The promise of Dochu is not merely technical—it represents a paradigm shift toward the *democratization of embolization*, making it accessible, scalable, and affordable.

Translating Catheter-Based Logic into a Simplified Procedure

How can we possibly replicate the sophistication of catheter-based embolization—a technique refined over five decades within interventional radiology—without fluoroscopy, without catheters, and without a dedicated angiography suite?

In traditional embolization, a catheter is inserted into a peripheral artery and skillfully navigated under fluoroscopic guidance toward a distant target. Once in position, an embolic agent is delivered to occlude pathological vessels. The idea that one could replicate similar outcomes by simply puncturing a superficial artery with a fine needle in an outpatient clinic may seem implausible at first.

But let us begin with a story—one that marked the genesis of this simplified approach.

In 2014, we were treating an 84-year-old woman suffering from severe thumb carpometacarpal (CMC) osteoarthritis. Our initial plan was to perform a transcatheter embolization, inserting a catheter via the right groin and advancing it to the radial artery that supplied her left hand. However, due to the patient's vascular tortuosity and the limited length of our available catheters, we could only reach the radial artery at the wrist level—far proximal to the actual inflammatory site.

With no alternative tools at hand, we decided to inject temporary embolic material from that more proximal site, hoping that it would reach the pathological neovasculature around the CMC joint. It was far from ideal, and we were concerned that our technical compromise might lead to suboptimal results.

Yet, 1 month later, the patient returned to clinic beaming with relief. Her symptoms had improved dramatically.

That moment was transformative. If injecting embolic agents from the radial artery at the wrist level could yield such clinical improvement, then perhaps we did not need to go through the groin at all. Perhaps we could access the artery directly at the wrist—where the pulse is palpable—under ultrasound guidance, and achieve the same effect without a catheter, without a wire, and without fluoroscopy.

We began developing and refining this concept, now known as Dochu. Over time, as results proved consistent, we formalized the technique and began publishing our findings.

In another case, a nationally ranked professional golfer came to us, on the verge of retiring due to persistent finger joint pain. We identified significant inflammation and planned a course of three embolization sessions. Because Dochu uses only a fine needle and syringe, it is cost-effective, minimally invasive, and safe to repeat. After three sessions, this patient returned to competition—pain-free.

Mimicking Catheter-Based Precision Without the Catheter

The essence of Dochu lies in emulating the effects of superselective embolization by identifying accessible arteries close to the target lesion and injecting embolic material under ultrasound guidance (Fig. 1.1). Although it lacks the pinpoint precision of microcatheter navigation, the treatment often delivers comparable therapeutic effects by covering a broader vascular territory that includes the pathological region.

For example, when treating elbow pain, the brachial artery is an ideal access point. However, direct injection into the brachial artery often results in most of the

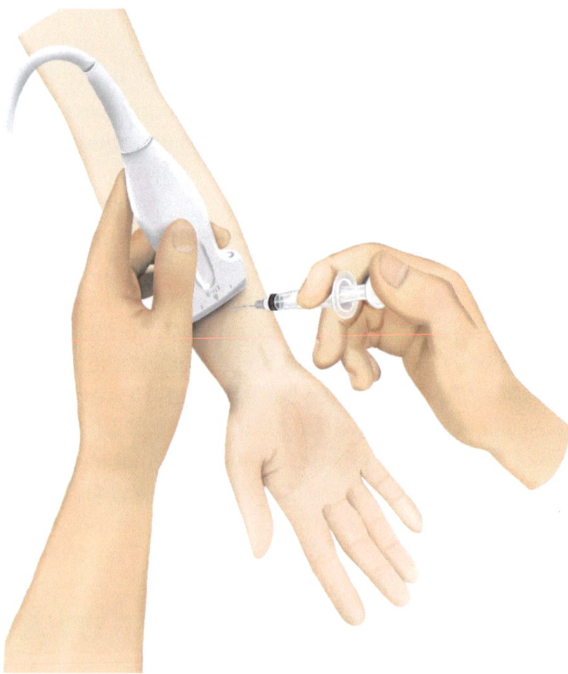

Fig. 1.1 Illustration of an ultrasound-guided puncture of the radial artery using a short-axis approach. (Illustrator: Misaki Kobayachi)

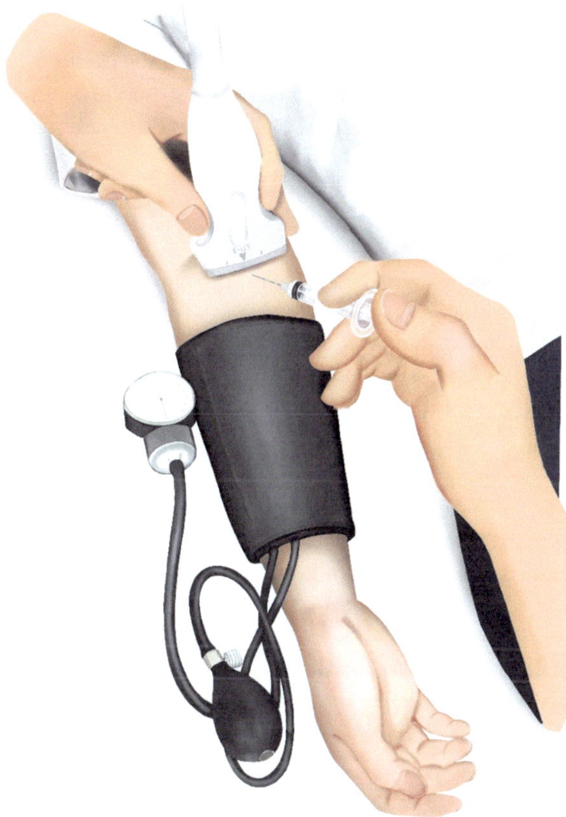

Fig. 1.2 Illustration of an ultrasound-guided puncture of the brachial artery performed under cuff compression to occlude distal flow. (Illustrator: Misaki Kobayachi)

embolic material flowing distally toward the fingers, rather than effectively reaching the target branches that supply the elbow. To address this, we use a simple blood pressure cuff on the forearm to reduce distal flow, redirecting the embolic agents into the inflamed branches supplying the elbow joint (Fig. 1.2).

Such flow control techniques using simple blood pressure cuffs are critical to the success of this method. They allow clinicians to adapt to anatomical challenges and maximize the delivery of embolic agents to the intended area.

Technical Considerations: Arterial Size, Tools, and Agents

The arteries targeted with Dochu must be large enough to permit safe and accurate needle access. From our experience, vessels smaller than 1.3 mm in diameter become technically difficult to puncture, with 1.4 mm or greater being preferable.

The procedure also benefits from a two-person technique. The operator holds the ultrasound probe and stabilizes the needle, while an assistant delivers the embolic agent through a syringe connected by a short, narrow extension tube. This prevents needle displacement during injection—a risk when working with small vessels.

Only *temporary embolic agents* should be used. Permanent agents are inappropriate in this context. The ideal embolic should be greater than 100 μm and less than 200 μm in diameter to minimize neurovascular risk and must dissolve within approximately 1 hour in healthy vasculature to prevent ischemic complications, especially if inadvertently delivered to distal arteries.

Appropriate Indications and Inappropriate Ones

Conditions suitable for Dochu typically share a pathophysiological profile: abnormal neovascularization, neurogenic inflammation, and chronic pain. This includes osteoarthritis, tendinopathy, adhesive capsulitis, synovitis, bursitis, gout, rheumatoid arthritis, and even early complex regional pain syndrome (CRPS). In these scenarios, reducing pathological vessels helps reset the inflammatory microenvironment and restore normal tissue dynamics.

However, the technique is *not effective* in cases where pain is purely mechanical (e.g., meniscal tears or impingement), psychogenic, or driven by central sensitization in chronic-stage CRPS. It also offers limited benefit when no inflammatory or neovascular component is evident.

What Have We Achieved So Far?

At the time of its inception, the concept of simplified intra-arterial embolization without fluoroscopy or catheters—administered through a fine needle under ultrasound guidance—seemed ambitious, if not implausible. Yet today, clinical evidence from multiple disease contexts confirms not only the feasibility of this approach but also its substantial clinical benefit and remarkable safety profile.

In patients with distal and proximal interphalangeal (DIP/PIP) joint osteoarthritis, a retrospective study of 92 cases showed a 77% clinical success rate at 12 months, with significant pain and functional improvement and no major complications.

A separate prospective study targeting trapeziometacarpal (TM) osteoarthritis reported similar results: 74% of patients achieved meaningful improvement at 24 months, with Numeric Rating Scale (NRS) pain scores dropping from 7.2 to 2.5. Many required no more than one or two treatments, and no serious adverse events were observed.

In plantar fasciitis, a condition known for treatment resistance, 66 patients underwent the same simplified approach via the posterior tibial artery. Pain scores improved from 7.9 to 0.7 at the final follow-up (~31 months), with functional scores increasing from 65.8 to 96.1. All adverse events were mild and temporary.

These results confirm several key principles of simplified intra-arterial embolization:

- *Reproducibility*: Across different joints and tendinous structures, the technique consistently delivers therapeutic benefit.

- *Safety*: Temporary embolic agents like IPM/CS allow rapid reperfusion in healthy vessels, minimizing the risk of ischemia.
- *Efficiency*: Most procedures are completed in under 3 minutes and performed in outpatient clinics without radiation exposure.
- *Repeatability*: The low invasiveness enables multiple treatments when needed, allowing sustained control of chronic pain.

While randomized controlled trials are still needed to establish comparative efficacy, these early results validate the therapeutic potential of Dochu. More than just an alternative to catheter-based embolization, it represents a paradigm shift—one that makes interventional logic accessible to a wider range of clinicians and patients.

The Power of Minimal Invasiveness and a Vision for Prevention

One of the most remarkable features of Dochu is its *extremely low invasiveness*. Puncturing a radial artery with a 27G needle rarely causes bleeding or visible trauma. The arterial wall heals rapidly, leaving no trace. This means the procedure can be *safely repeated*, which opens new clinical possibilities.

In osteoarthritis, for example, it is well known that synovitis fuels structural degeneration. With a conventional catheter-based embolization, early intervention is limited by cost and invasiveness. But Dochu may allow early and repeated interventions—even in patients in their 30s and 40s—to suppress inflammation and potentially slow or halt disease progression. While this is still a hypothesis requiring long-term study, it is a vision worth pursuing.

Opening a New Door

Dochu is not a replacement for interventional radiology—it is an expansion of its philosophy. By stripping embolization down to its essential components and reimagining its delivery, we offer a new tool to a wider community of clinicians.

This book aims to equip you with the knowledge, confidence, and practical skills to perform Dochu safely and effectively. The following chapters will walk you through each target condition, step-by-step, from anatomy to ultrasound guidance to embolic selection.

We are at the beginning of a new chapter in pain intervention—one that is simpler, safer, and more accessible.

Let us begin.

2 Neck and Upper Extremity

Trapezius Muscle Pain/Neck Pain

Introduction

Trapezius muscle pain is a prevalent musculoskeletal condition that affects the large trapezius muscle, which spans the neck, shoulders, and upper back. This type of pain is often caused by muscle strain, tension, or overuse, and is a frequent contributor to neck pain. The discomfort associated with trapezius muscle pain can vary from mild stiffness to severe, debilitating pain that interferes with daily activities and mobility [1, 2].

Epidemiology

Neck pain and trapezius muscle pain are widespread conditions that affect both sedentary and active populations. It is estimated that up to 30% of adults experience neck pain annually, with trapezius muscle pain being a leading cause of discomfort, particularly in office workers and individuals with physically demanding jobs. These conditions are common across all age groups but occur most frequently in individuals aged 20 to 50 years. Women and those with poor posture or sedentary lifestyles are particularly susceptible. Risk factors include poor posture, especially during prolonged desk work or screen use, muscle overuse or repetitive activities such as carrying heavy loads or engaging in sports, stress and anxiety that contribute to muscle tension, and inadequate ergonomics in work or home environments [3–5].

Y. Okuno et al., *Ultrasound-guided Musculoskeletal Embolotherapies using the "Dochu" Technique*, https://doi.org/10.1007/978-3-032-17250-1_2

Clinical Presentation and Symptoms

Patients with trapezius muscle pain or neck pain often report a variety of symptoms. Pain is typically described as dull and aching, localized to the trapezius muscle or the base of the neck. In severe cases, the pain may radiate to the shoulders, upper back, or arms. Symptoms often worsen with prolonged sitting, standing, or specific activities like lifting. Muscle stiffness is a common complaint, particularly after waking or long periods of inactivity [6, 7].

Palpable tenderness or knots, also known as myofascial trigger points, are frequently found in the trapezius muscle. Patients may also experience a reduced range of motion, making it difficult to turn the head, tilt the neck, or raise the arms overhead. Functional limitations, such as discomfort during daily activities like driving, working at a computer, or exercising, are common. Associated symptoms may include headaches originating from muscle tension (tension-type headaches) and a sensation of fatigue or heaviness in the shoulders [8].

Pathophysiology

The causes of trapezius muscle pain involve mechanical stress, inflammation, and neuromuscular dysfunction. Repetitive activities or sustained positions can lead to muscle overuse and strain, causing microtrauma in muscle fibers. The accumulation of metabolic by-products such as lactic acid exacerbates pain and stiffness. Myofascial trigger points often develop due to localized muscle tension, resulting in referred pain [9, 10].

Postural imbalances, such as forward head posture or slouched shoulders, place excessive strain on the trapezius muscle, leading to chronic tension. Muscle irritation can trigger a localized inflammatory response, causing swelling and discomfort. Neurological contributions include the hyperactivation of sensory nerves due to muscle tension, which sensitizes pain pathways. Psychological stress further exacerbates the condition by increasing sympathetic nervous system activity, resulting in sustained muscle contraction [11, 12].

Treatment Options

Management of trapezius muscle pain focuses on relieving pain, improving posture, and preventing recurrence [13–18]:

- *Non-pharmacological:*
  - *Physical Therapy*:
    Stretching exercises for the neck, shoulders, and upper back to reduce tension
    Strengthening exercises for postural muscles, such as the rhomboids and core
    Massage therapy to alleviate trigger points and improve circulation

  - *Postural Correction*:
    Ergonomic adjustments in the workplace, including chair and desk setup
    Encouraging proper posture during daily activities
  - *Heat or Ice Therapy*:
    Heat packs to relax muscle tension or ice packs to reduce inflammation
  - *Stress Management:*
    Relaxation techniques such as deep breathing, yoga, or mindfulness to reduce tension
  - *Acupuncture or Dry Needling*:
    Targeting myofascial trigger points for pain relief and muscle relaxation
- *Pharmacological:*
  - *NSAIDs or acetaminophen for short-term pain relief*
  - *Muscle relaxants for severe muscle spasms*
  - *Topical analgesics, such as menthol or capsaicin creams, for localized pain management*
- *Procedural/Surgical:*
  - *Trigger Point Injections*:
    Local anesthetics or corticosteroids to alleviate chronic muscle tension
  - *Botulinum Toxin (Botox) Injections*:
    For persistent muscle tightness or spasm
  - *Rarely, surgical interventions may be required for underlying structural abnormalities.*
- *Emerging Tvherapies:*
  - Platelet-rich plasma (PRP) injections for muscle repair
  - Electrical stimulation or ultrasound therapy to promote muscle relaxation and healing

In conclusion, trapezius muscle pain and neck pain are common conditions that can significantly affect daily life. Addressing the underlying causes, such as poor posture or stress, through conservative measures like physical therapy and ergonomic adjustments, is essential for effective management. For chronic or severe cases, advanced treatments such as trigger point injections or emerging therapies can provide relief and restore function.

Dochu algorithm: trapezius muscle pain (neck pain)	
External landmarks	Palpable supraclavicular fossa
Probe positioning	Probe orientation nearly perpendicular to the clavicle The initial position of the ultrasound probe should be nearly parallel to the clavicle. This orientation allows for an optimal view of the relevant anatomical structures, including the anterior scalene muscle, the brachial plexus, and the middle scalene muscle. Then rotate the probe 90 degrees so that it is perpendicular to the clavicle (Fig. 2.1). This step is essential for confirming the anatomy and ensuring that the puncture site avoids critical neurovascular structures

(continued)

Target vessel	Transverse cervical artery (Fig. 2.2 and 2.3)
Needle size	27G length: 25 mm
Medication	Imipenem/Cilastatin (1 vial: 0.5 g/0.5 g) diluted with 10 cc of saline
Dosage	2–3 ml
Cuff position	NA

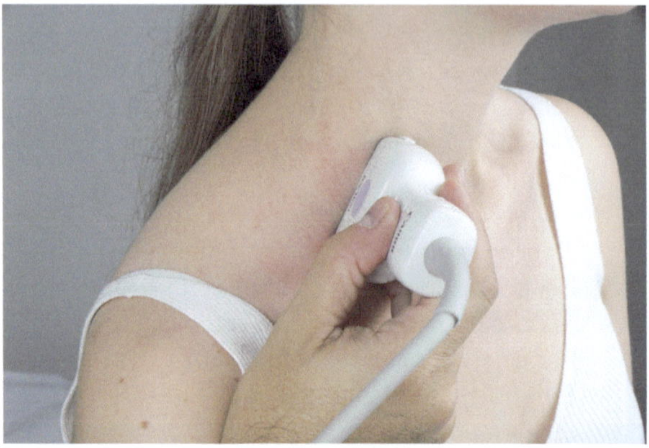

Fig. 2.1 Probe orientation nearly perpendiclar to the clavicle at the level of the supraclavicular fossa

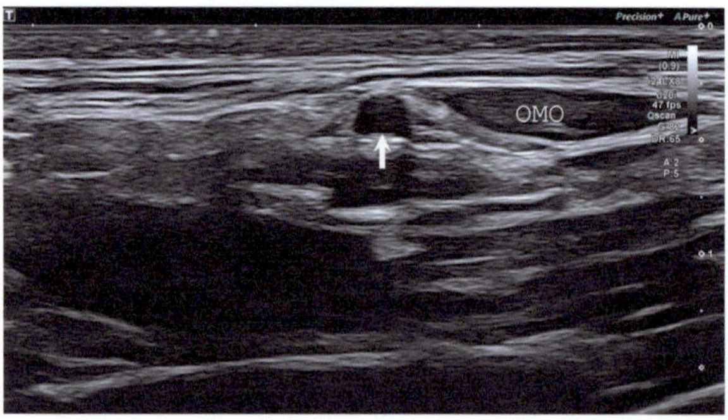

Fig. 2.2 Depiction of the transverse cervical artery (arrow) in near proximity to the inferior belly of the omohyoid muscle (OMO)

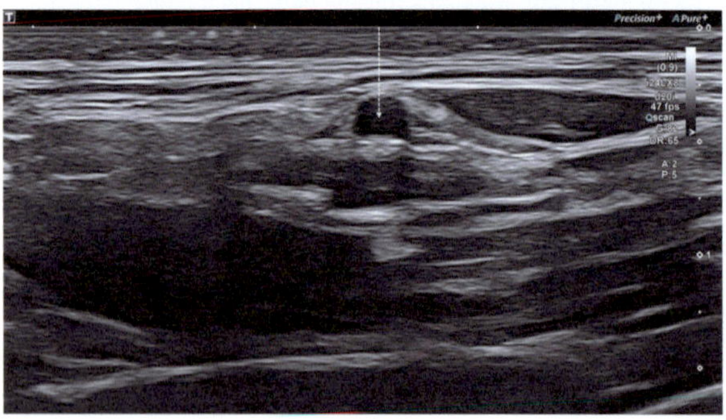

Fig. 2.3 Needle entry path in an "out-of-plane access" (dotted arrow)

Shoulder Stiffness/Shoulder Osteoarthritis (OA)

Introduction

Shoulder osteoarthritis (OA) is a degenerative joint condition affecting the glenohumeral joint, characterized by progressive cartilage loss, pain, stiffness, and reduced mobility. While it is less common than osteoarthritis of the knee or hip, it has a significant impact on quality of life due to the essential role of the shoulder in daily activities. The condition typically develops as a result of age-related wear and tear, but it can also occur secondary to trauma, rotator cuff injuries, or inflammatory diseases [19, 20].

Epidemiology

Shoulder OA is most prevalent in older adults, although secondary forms of the condition can affect younger individuals. It is estimated that approximately 4% of adults over the age of 60 experience shoulder OA. The condition is commonly seen in individuals over 50, with prevalence increasing with age. Several risk factors contribute to its development, including a history of shoulder trauma, such as fractures or dislocations, and repetitive overhead activities, which are often associated with sports or manual labor. Rotator cuff tears, particularly those leading to cuff tear arthropathy, can also result in OA. Other contributing factors include a genetic predisposition or family history of osteoarthritis, as well as systemic inflammatory conditions such as rheumatoid arthritis [20–22].

Clinical Presentation and Symptoms

Patients with shoulder OA often report a combination of pain, stiffness, and functional limitations. Pain is typically described as a deep, aching sensation localized to the shoulder, which is worsened by activities such as overhead movements, lifting, or reaching behind the back. In advanced stages, pain may occur at rest or during the night, leading to disrupted sleep. Stiffness usually develops gradually, resulting in a reduced range of motion, particularly in external rotation and abduction. This can make everyday tasks such as dressing, combing hair, or reaching overhead increasingly difficult [23, 24].

Crepitus, characterized by grinding, clicking, or popping sensations during shoulder movement, is another common symptom caused by bone-on-bone contact or the presence of osteophytes. Mild swelling and tenderness around the joint may also occur, with tenderness most pronounced upon palpation of the anterior shoulder. Functional limitations, such as reduced ability to perform work or recreational activities involving the shoulder and a loss of strength in advanced cases, can significantly affect a patient's quality of life [23, 24].

Pathophysiology

Shoulder OA is defined by progressive cartilage degeneration, joint remodeling, and inflammation. The loss of articular cartilage covering the humeral head and glenoid leads to bone-on-bone friction, triggering synovial inflammation as cartilage breakdown products accumulate. Osteophytes, or bone spurs, form at joint margins as the body attempts to stabilize the joint, further restricting movement and contributing to pain [19, 25].

Chronic cartilage loss results in joint space narrowing, increasing mechanical stress, while hypervascularity in the synovium exacerbates swelling and pain as part of the body's repair attempts. Subchondral bone changes, including sclerosis and the formation of cysts, also occur due to stress and remodeling. These pathological changes collectively lead to the characteristic symptoms of shoulder OA, including pain, stiffness, and reduced function [19, 25].

Treatment Options

Treatment of shoulder OA aims to reduce pain, restore function, and prevent further degeneration [19, 20, 25–27]:

- *Non-pharmacological*:
  - Physical therapy focusing on improving range of motion, strength, and posture
  - Heat or ice therapy to manage pain and stiffness
  - Activity modification to avoid aggravating movements
  - Use of supportive devices like slings during flare-ups
- *Pharmacological*:
  - NSAIDs for pain relief and inflammation control
  - Topical analgesics for localized symptom management
  - Corticosteroid injections for temporary relief of inflammation and severe pain
  - Hyaluronic acid injections to improve joint lubrication (limited evidence for the shoulder compared to knee OA)
- *Procedural/Surgical*:
  - Arthroscopic debridement to remove loose cartilage or bone fragments
  - Shoulder joint replacement (total shoulder arthroplasty or reverse shoulder arthroplasty) in advanced cases with significant pain and disability
  - Hemiarthroplasty for isolated humeral head degeneration
- *Emerging Therapies*:
  - Platelet-rich plasma (PRP) or stem cell injections for cartilage repair and inflammation reduction
  - Biologic therapies targeting inflammatory cytokines in systemic conditions

In conclusion, shoulder OA is a challenging condition that significantly impacts patients' mobility and quality of life. Early diagnosis and a multidisciplinary approach, combining conservative treatments with advanced surgical and regenerative options, can effectively manage symptoms and improve outcomes for those affected by this debilitating condition.

Dochu algorithm: shoulder osteoarthritis/adhesive capsulitis	
External landmarks	Ventral axillary fold, palpable pulsation of the axillary artery
Probe positioning	Transverse oblique probe orientation at the ventral axillary fold (Fig. 2.4) ensures optimal visualization of the axillary artery proximal to the origin of the posterior circumflex humeral artery
Target vessel	Axillary artery (Fig. 2.5 and 2.6)
Needle size	27G, length: 25–38 mm
Medication	Imipenem/Cilastatin (1 vial: 0.5 g/0.5 g) diluted with 10 cc of saline
Dosage	3 ml
Cuff position	Upper arm
Cuff compression duration	Deflate cuff 30 s after injection

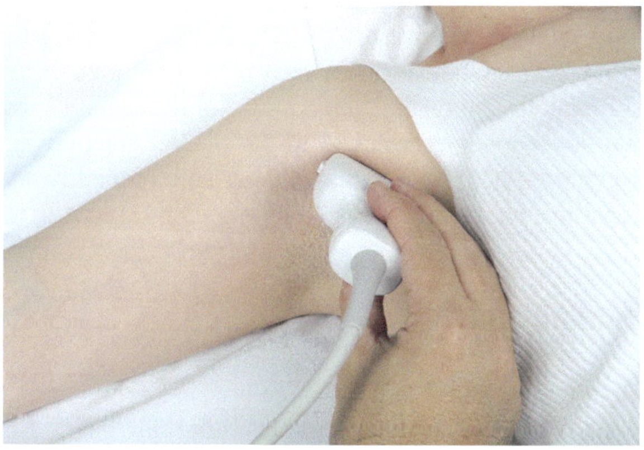

Fig. 2.4 Longitudinal probe orientation at the ventral axillary fold, transverse oblique to the course of the extended upper arm

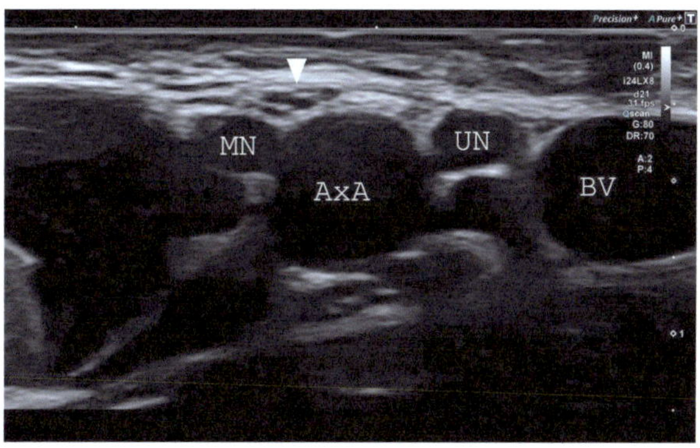

Fig. 2.5 Depiction of the axillary artery (AxA) between the hypoechogenic median nerve (MN) and ulnar nerve (UN). Cave: Medial cutaneous antebrachial nerve (arrowhead) lying superficial to the axillary artery. Basilic vein (BV)

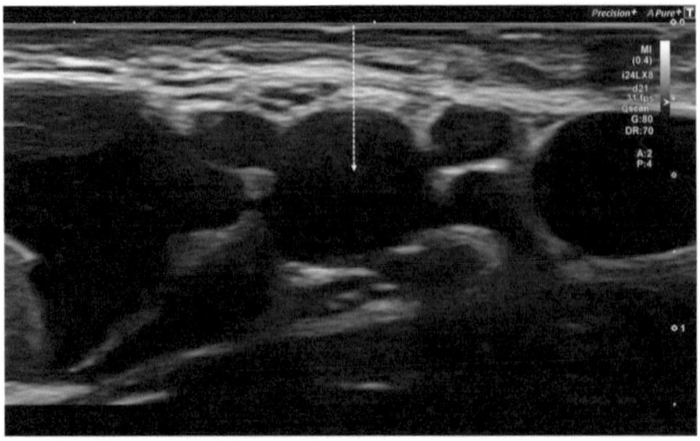

Fig. 2.6 Needle entry path in an out of plane access (dotted arrow) ulnar to the medical cutaneous antebrachial nerve

Tennis Elbow (Lateral Epicondylitis) and Golfer's Elbow (Medial Epicondylitis)

Introduction

Tennis elbow, also known as lateral epicondylitis, and golfer's elbow, or medial epicondylitis, are overuse injuries caused by repetitive strain on the forearm tendons. Tennis elbow is characterized by inflammation and degeneration of the extensor tendons at the lateral epicondyle of the humerus, whereas golfer's elbow affects the flexor tendons attached to the medial epicondyle. Despite their names, these conditions are not limited to athletes and frequently occur in individuals engaged in repetitive wrist and forearm motions [28–32].

Epidemiology

Both tennis elbow and golfer's elbow are common conditions, particularly in individuals aged 30 to 50, and share similar risk factors. Tennis elbow affects approximately 1–3% of adults annually, with a higher incidence among individuals who perform repetitive wrist extension [33–35]. In contrast, golfer's elbow is less prevalent, affecting about 0.4–0.6% of adults [35]. Risk factors for both conditions include repetitive wrist and forearm movements such as gripping, lifting, or twisting, as well as occupations like carpentry, painting, or prolonged computer use. In sports, poor technique or inappropriate equipment can increase the risk, and weak forearm muscles or inadequate conditioning further exacerbates susceptibility [28–30, 34, 35].

Clinical Presentation and Symptoms

The clinical presentations of tennis elbow and golfer's elbow overlap but are distinguished by the specific tendons involved.

Tennis elbow presents with pain and tenderness over the lateral epicondyle, often radiating down the forearm. This pain is exacerbated by gripping or lifting objects and can lead to weakness in wrist extension, making tasks such as opening jars or shaking hands difficult. Symptoms are typically aggravated by activities that involve repetitive wrist extension [30, 33].

Golfer's elbow, on the other hand, is characterized by pain and tenderness over the medial epicondyle, with pain radiating along the inner forearm. Patients may experience weakness in wrist flexion and grip strength, and symptoms worsen during activities requiring repetitive wrist flexion or pronation, such as swinging a golf club or lifting heavy objects [32, 36].

Pathophysiology

Both conditions are the result of repetitive microtrauma and overuse of the tendons attached to the epicondyles of the humerus. Repeated stress leads to microscopic tears in the tendon fibers, which initiate an inflammatory response. Persistent strain disrupts the natural healing process, resulting in tendinosis, a degenerative condition without significant inflammation. Hypervascularity, or neovascularization, often develops in the affected tendons, contributing to pain and impaired function. Mechanical overload from repetitive motions and inadequate recovery further exacerbates the damage, leading to tendon degeneration and chronic symptoms [37, 38].

Treatment Options

Management focuses on pain relief, promoting tendon healing, and preventing recurrence [38–43]:

- *Non pharmacological*:
  - Rest and activity modification to avoid repetitive strain
  - Application of ice packs to reduce pain and inflammation
  - Physical therapy:
    Eccentric strengthening exercises for tendon repair
    Stretching exercises for flexibility and reduced tension
  - Use of braces or counterforce straps to offload the affected tendon
  - Ergonomic adjustments for workplace or sports activities
- *Pharmacological*:
  - NSAIDs for pain and inflammation management in the acute phase
  - Topical anti-inflammatory agents for localized symptom control
  - Corticosteroid injections for temporary relief in severe cases, though they may delay tendon healing
- *Procedural/Surgical*:
  - Percutaneous needle tenotomy to stimulate tissue repair
  - Platelet-rich plasma (PRP) injections to promote tendon regeneration

  - Surgical debridement for chronic cases unresponsive to conservative treatment
- *Emerging Therapies*:
  - Shockwave therapy to stimulate tissue healing
  - Stem cell therapy for tendon repair and regeneration
  - Biologics targeting inflammatory pathways in chronic tendinosis

In conclusion, tennis elbow and golfer's elbow are debilitating overuse injuries that can significantly impair hand and arm function. Early diagnosis, activity modification, and structured rehabilitation programs are key to effective recovery. For persistent cases, advanced therapies such as PRP and shockwave therapy provide promising options for tendon healing and long-term symptom relief.

Dochu algorithm: tennis elbow/Golfers elbow	
External landmarks	Palpation of the pulsating brachial artery at the level of the medial humeral epicondyle
Probe positioning	Transverse oblique probe orientation between the medial humeral epicondyle and the biceps brachii tendon is used to accurately identify the brachial artery (Fig. 2.7)
Target vessel	Brachial artery (Fig. 2.8 and 2.9)
Needle size	27G, length: 19 mm
Medication	Imipenem/Cilastatin (1vial: 0.5 g/0.5 g) diluted with 10 cc of saline
Dosage	2 ml
Cuff position	Forearm
Cuff compression duration	Deflate cuff 10 s after injection

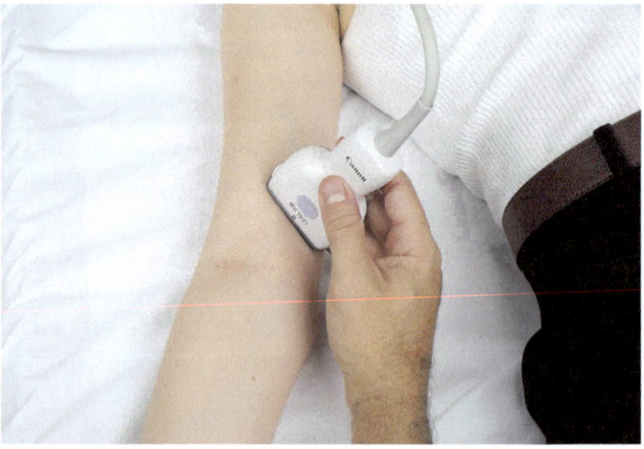

Fig. 2.7 Positioning of the probe between the palpable medial epicondyle and the medial distal biceps tendon in a transverse oblique orientation

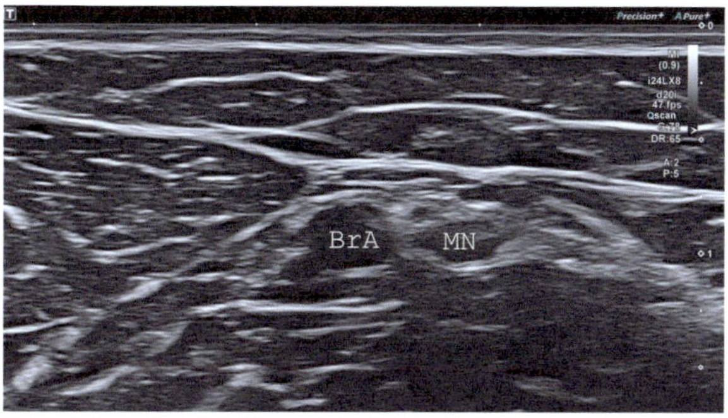

Fig. 2.8 Depiction of the brachial artery (BrA) mostly found immediately radial to the median nerve (MN)

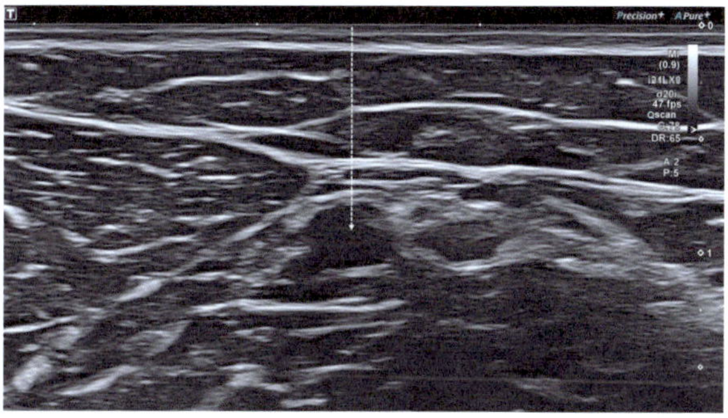

Fig. 2.9 Needle entry path in an out-of-plane access (dotted arrow). Cave: median nerve!

De Quervain's Tenosynovitis

Introduction

De Quervain's tenosynovitis is a painful condition resulting from inflammation of the tendons in the first dorsal compartment of the wrist, specifically the abductor pollicis longus (APL) and extensor pollicis brevis (EPB). It is commonly associated with repetitive thumb and wrist movements, causing pain and swelling near the base of the thumb. Often referred to as "mommy thumb" due to its prevalence among new parents, this condition can significantly impact hand function and daily activities [44, 45].

Epidemiology

De Quervain's tenosynovitis is a relatively common condition, particularly in populations that engage in repetitive hand and wrist use. It is more prevalent in women, especially those aged 30 to 50 years and frequently occurs in individuals with occupations or hobbies that involve repetitive thumb or wrist motions, such as musicians, athletes, and office workers [44, 46]. Key risk factors include repetitive activities involving the thumb and wrist, such as lifting, gripping, or texting, as well as pregnancy and the postpartum period due to hormonal changes and increased wrist strain. Trauma or direct injury to the wrist and underlying inflammatory conditions, such as rheumatoid arthritis, also contribute to its development [46, 47].

Clinical Presentation and Symptoms

Patients with De Quervain's tenosynovitis typically present with distinct symptoms localized to the thumb and wrist. Pain is often the primary complaint, located on the radial side of the wrist near the base of the thumb. This pain worsens with thumb movement or activities such as gripping, pinching, or twisting and may radiate into the forearm or thumb. Visible swelling over the first dorsal compartment of the wrist is common, and patients may experience stiffness or difficulty moving the thumb or wrist, particularly in the morning or after periods of rest [44, 48, 49].

Tenderness is often noted on palpation of the affected tendons near the radial styloid, and some patients report crepitus—a grinding or creaking sensation during tendon movement. Functional limitations, such as difficulty performing tasks that require thumb and wrist coordination, including holding objects, opening jars, or typing, are frequently observed [44, 49, 58].

Pathophysiology

De Quervain's tenosynovitis develops as a result of mechanical irritation and inflammation of the APL and EPB tendons. Repetitive thumb movements cause friction and irritation of the tendons within the narrow fibro-osseous tunnel of the first dorsal compartment. This leads to the inflammation of the synovial lining, causing swelling, pain, and restricted tendon gliding. Hypervascularity, or increased vascular proliferation, occurs as part of the inflammatory response, contributing to tenderness and swelling. Chronic irritation can result in fibrosis, with thickening of the tendon sheath and the formation of scar tissue, further limiting tendon movement [44, 49].

Treatment Options

Treatment for De Quervain's tenosynovitis focuses on reducing inflammation, alleviating pain, and restoring hand function [44, 48, 50–54]:

- *Non-Pharmacological*:
  - *Rest and Activity Modification*:
    Avoid repetitive thumb and wrist movements that exacerbate symptoms.
    Modify daily activities or workplace ergonomics to reduce strain.

  - *Immobilization*:
    Use of a thumb spica splint to support the wrist and thumb, allowing tendons to rest and heal.
  - *Physical Therapy*:
    Stretching and strengthening exercises for the wrist and thumb
    Ultrasound therapy to reduce inflammation and promote healing
  - *Ergonomic Adjustments*:
    Use of adaptive tools or braces for repetitive tasks
- *Pharmacological*:
  - NSAIDs for pain relief and inflammation control
  - Topical analgesics for localized pain management
  - Corticosteroid injections into the first dorsal compartment for significant swelling or pain relief
- *Procedural/Surgical*:
  - *Surgical Decompression*:
    Release of the first dorsal compartment to relieve tendon entrapment in refractory cases
  - *Percutaneous Release*:
    Minimally invasive procedure to cut the retinaculum and allow tendon gliding
- *Emerging Therapies*:
  - Platelet-rich plasma (PRP) injections to reduce inflammation and promote tendon repair
  - Biologic therapies targeting inflammatory cytokines

In conclusion, De Quervain's tenosynovitis is a common overuse injury that can significantly impact hand and wrist function. Early diagnosis and conservative management with rest, splinting, and physical therapy are often effective. For chronic or refractory cases, advanced treatments, including corticosteroid injections or surgical release, can provide long-term relief and restore functionality.

Dochu algorithm: De-Quervains tenosynovitis	
External landmarks	1. Palpate the radial artery at the distal lower arm
Probe positioning	1. Transverse probe orientation approx. 5 cm proximal to the carpal crease over the radial artery (Fig. 2.10)
Target vessel	Radial artery (Figs. 2.11 and 2.12)
Needle size	27G, length: 19 mm
Medication	Imipenem/Cilastatin (1 vial: 0.5 g/0.5 g) diluted with 10 cc of saline
Dosage	1 ml
Cuff position	Hand
Cuff compression duration	Deflate cuff 30 s after injection

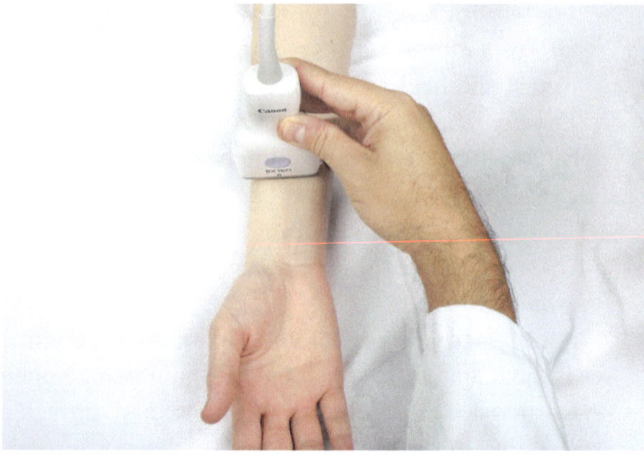

Fig. 2.10 Transverse probe orientation at the distal forearm (approx. 5 cm proximal to the carpal crease) over the palpable radial artery

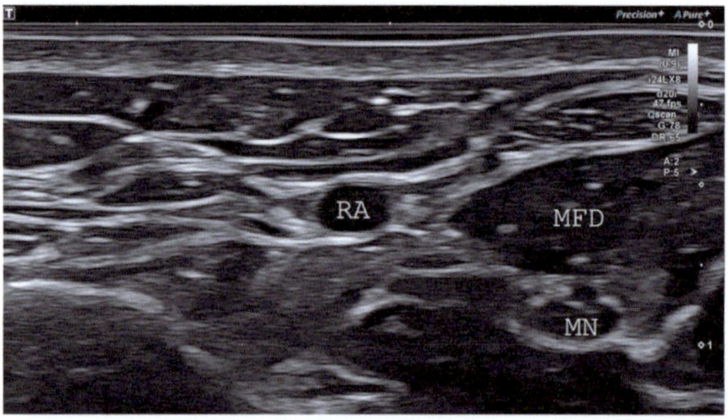

Fig. 2.11 Depiction of the radial artery (RA) at the level of the distal forearm, radial to the Flexor digitorum muscles (MFD) and the median nerve (MN)

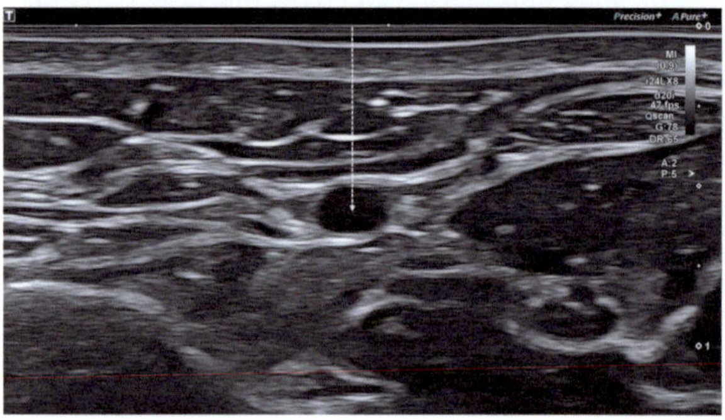

Fig. 2.12 Needle entry path in an out of plane access (dotted arrow)

Rheumatoid Arthritis (RA)—Wrist and Finger

Introduction

Rheumatoid arthritis (RA) is a chronic systemic autoimmune disorder that primarily affects synovial joints, causing inflammation, pain, and progressive joint destruction. Unlike osteoarthritis, which is a degenerative condition, RA is an inflammatory disease characterized by immune-mediated damage. In addition to joint involvement, RA can affect extra-articular tissues, including the skin, heart, lungs, and eyes, making it a multi-systemic disease [55–57].

Epidemiology

RA affects millions of people worldwide and demonstrates specific demographic patterns. It has a prevalence of approximately 0.5–1% globally and is more common in women, with a female-to-male ratio of 3:1. The condition typically presents between the ages of 30 and 60 but can occur at any age. Risk factors for RA include a genetic predisposition, particularly associated with the HLA-DR4 and HLA-DR1 alleles, and environmental triggers such as smoking, which is a significant risk factor. Hormonal influences contribute to its higher prevalence in women, and infections may also play a role in triggering autoimmune activity [58–60].

Clinical Presentation and Symptoms

RA usually has an insidious onset, involving multiple joints and potentially progressing to systemic manifestations. Articular symptoms include symmetric joint pain and swelling, most commonly affecting the small joints of the hands, wrists, and feet. Patients often experience morning stiffness lasting longer than 30 minutes, as well as warmth, redness, and tenderness over affected joints. Without treatment, the condition can lead to progressive joint deformities, such as ulnar deviation, swan neck deformities, or boutonnière deformities [61–63].

Systemic symptoms may include fatigue, fever, malaise, loss of appetite, and unintended weight loss. Extra-articular manifestations are common and may include rheumatoid nodules, which are firm, subcutaneous nodules over pressure points. Pulmonary involvement can manifest as interstitial lung disease or pleural effusion, while cardiovascular complications may include pericarditis and an increased risk of atherosclerosis. Ocular manifestations such as scleritis or keratoconjunctivitis sicca and vasculitis leading to skin ulcers or peripheral neuropathy are also observed in some cases [61–64].

Pathophysiology

RA is an autoimmune disease driven by immune system dysregulation and persistent synovial inflammation. Environmental or genetic triggers activate autoreactive T cells and B cells, with the latter producing autoantibodies such as rheumatoid factor (RF) and anti-citrullinated protein antibodies (ACPAs). These immune responses lead to the infiltration of activated immune cells into the synovium, releasing pro-inflammatory cytokines such as tumor necrosis factor-alpha (TNF-α), interleukin-1 (IL-1), and interleukin-6 (IL-6) [65–67].

This inflammatory activity causes synovial hyperplasia, forming pannus tissue that invades and damages cartilage and bone. Osteoclast activation contributes to bone erosion, while matrix metalloproteinases (MMPs) degrade cartilage. Systemic inflammation is driven by elevated levels of cytokines and acute-phase reactants such as C-reactive protein (CRP), contributing to systemic symptoms. Hypervascularity within the synovium sustains the inflammatory process and promotes pannus formation [65, 66].

Treatment Options

Management of RA involves controlling inflammation, preventing joint damage, and maintaining function [56, 68–72]:

- *Non-Pharmacological*:
  - *Physical Therapy*:
    Exercises to maintain joint flexibility and muscle strength
    Splinting or bracing to support affected joints
  - *Occupational Therapy*:
    Adaptive devices to assist with daily activities
    Ergonomic modifications to reduce joint strain
  - *Lifestyle Modifications*:
    Smoking cessation to reduce disease progression
    Balanced diet and regular exercise to improve overall health
- *Pharmacological*:
  - *Nonsteroidal Anti-Inflammatory Drugs (NSAIDs)*:
    Provide pain relief and reduce inflammation but do not alter disease progression
  - *Corticosteroids*:
    Low-dose prednisone for acute flares or bridging therapy
  - *Disease-Modifying Antirheumatic Drugs (DMARDs)*:
    Methotrexate (first-line therapy) to slow disease progression
    Leflunomide, sulfasalazine, or hydroxychloroquine as alternatives or adjuncts
  - *Biologic DMARDs*:
    TNF inhibitors (e.g., etanercept, adalimumab) for refractory or severe disease
    IL-6 inhibitors (e.g., tocilizumab) or B-cell depletion therapy (e.g., rituximab) for targeted intervention.
  - *JAK Inhibitors*:
    Oral agents like tofacitinib for patients unresponsive to traditional DMARDs
- *Procedural/Surgical*:
  - *Joint Aspiration*:
    For relief of joint effusion and diagnostic evaluation
  - *Synovectomy*:
    Surgical removal of inflamed synovium in refractory cases
  - *Joint Replacement Surgery*:
    Total joint arthroplasty for severely damaged joints

- *Emerging Therapies*:
  - Targeted small molecules addressing specific inflammatory pathways
  - Precision medicine approaches leveraging genetic and biomarker profiling

In conclusion, RA is a complex autoimmune disease with significant potential for joint destruction and systemic complications. Early diagnosis and aggressive treatment using a combination of DMARDs, biologics, and supportive therapies can improve outcomes, slow disease progression, and enhance quality of life. Advances in immunomodulatory therapies offer promising avenues for achieving sustained remission in patients with RA.

Dochu algorithm: rheumatoid arthritis (wrist and finger)	
External landmarks	1. Palpate the radial artery at the distal lower arm 2. Palpate the ulnar artery at the distal lower arm 3. Palpate the pulsating brachial artery at the level of the medial humeral epicondyle (in cases where the above 1 and 2 cannot be achieved)
Probe positioning	1. Transverse probe orientation at the carpal crease over the radial artery (Fig. 2.13) 2. Transverse probe orientation at the carpal crease over the ulnar artery (Fig. 2.14) 3. Transverse oblique probe orientation between the medial humeral epicondyle and the biceps brachii tendon (in cases where the above 1 and 2 cannot be achieved) (Fig. 2.15)
Target vessel	1. Radial artery (Figs. 2.16 and 2.17) 2. Ulnar artery (Figs. 2.18 and 2.19) 3. Brachial artery (Figs. 2.20 and 2.21)
Needle size	27G, length: 19 mm
Medication	Imipenem/Cilastatin (1 vial: 0.5 g/0.5 g) diluted with 10 cc of saline
Dosage	1 ml each, 2 ml from the brachial artery
Cuff position	Hand (Note: the cuff may be applied when treating the wrist, but should not be used when treating the fingers)
Cuff compression duration	Deflate cuff 30 s after injection

*Dochu is performed on both arteries. In cases where the puncturing of the radial and ulnar artery cannot be achieved, Dochu can be performed on the brachial artery

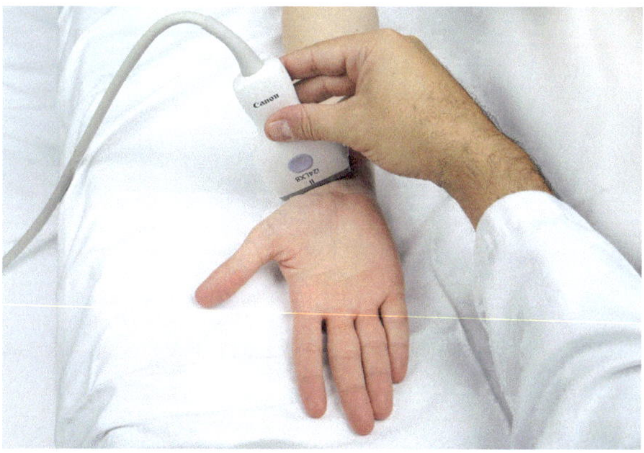

Fig. 2.13 Transverse probe orientation approx. 1 cm proximal to the carpal crease over the palpable radial artery

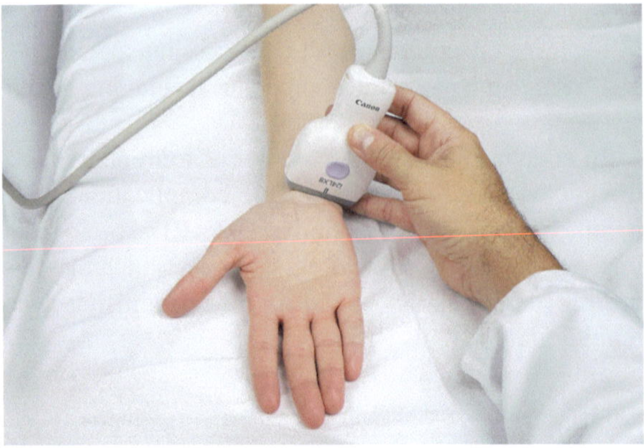

Fig. 2.14 Transverse probe orientation approx. 1 cm proximal to the carpal crease over the palpable ulnar artery

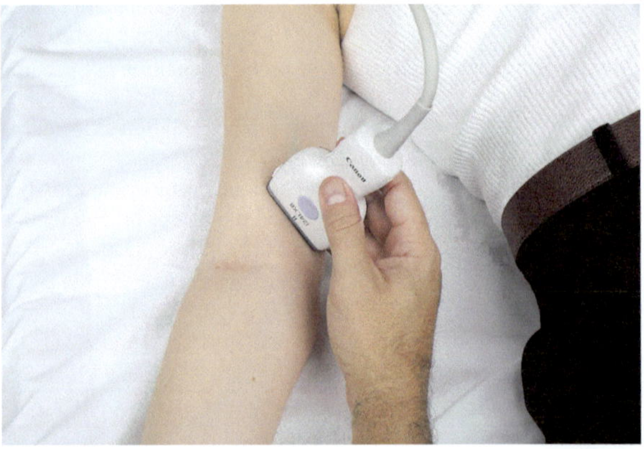

Fig. 2.15 Positioning of the probe between the palpable medial epicondyle and the medial distal biceps tendon in a transverse oblique orientation

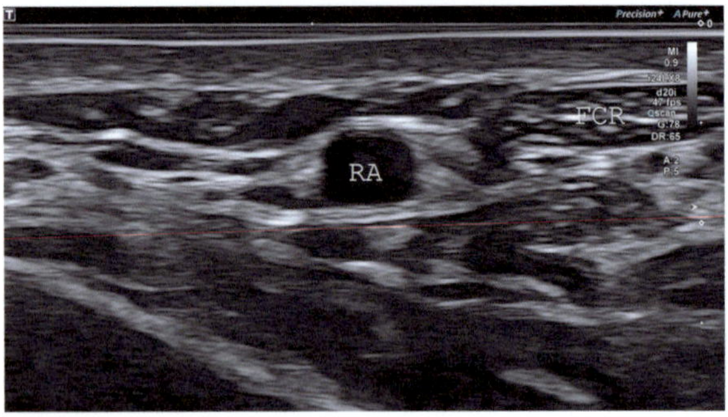

Fig. 2.16 Depiction of the radial artery (RA) at the level of the wrist radial to the flexor carpi radialis tendon (FCR)

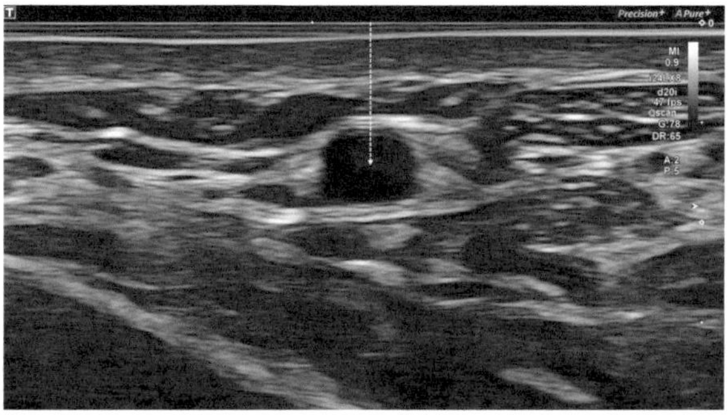

Fig. 2.17 Needle entry path in an out-of-plane access (dotted arrow)

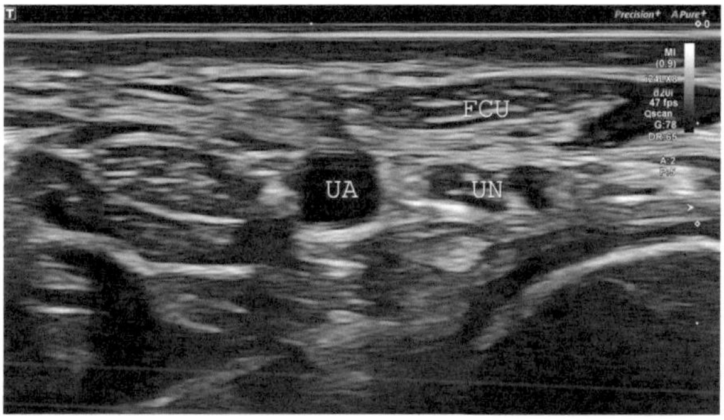

Fig. 2.18 Depiction of the ulnar artery (UA) radial to the ulnar nerve (UN) which is covered by the flecor carpi ulnaris tendon (FCU)

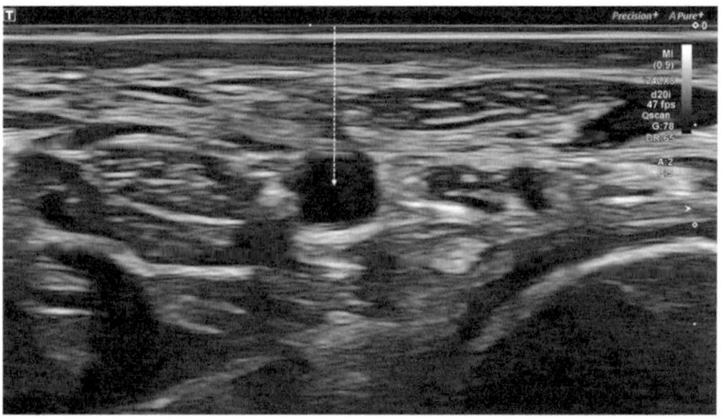

Fig. 2.19 Needle entry path in an out-of-plane access (dotted arrow). Cave: ulnar nerve!

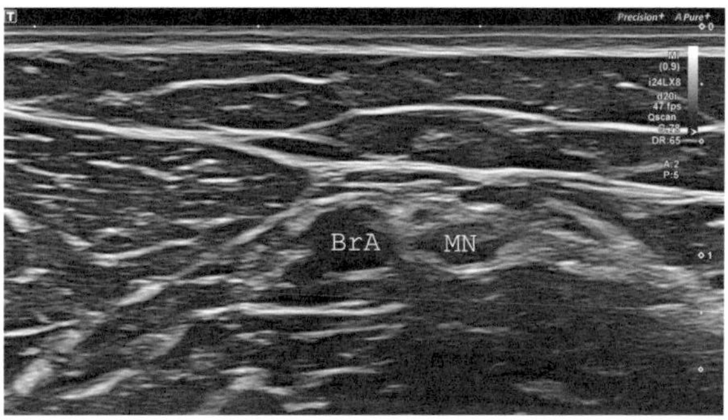

Fig. 2.20 Depiction of the brachial artery (BrA) mostly found immediately radial to the median nerve (MN)

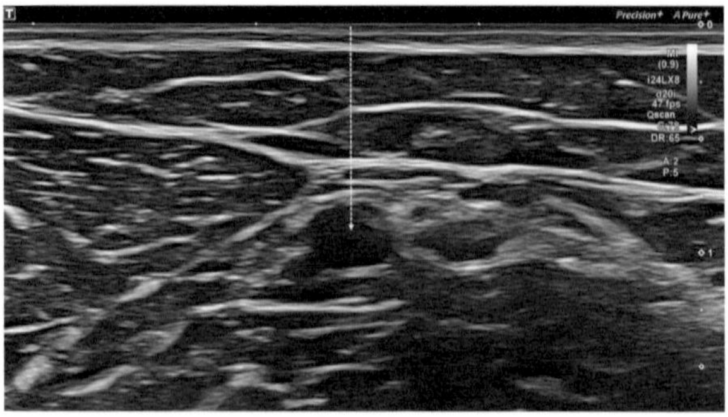

Fig. 2.21 Needle entry path in an out-of-plane access (dotted arrow). Cave: median nerve!

Carpometacarpal (CMC) Joint Arthritis and First CMC

Introduction

Carpometacarpal (CMC) joint arthritis, particularly of the first CMC joint (also known as thumb arthritis), is a common degenerative condition that affects the joint where the base of the thumb meets the wrist. This joint is critical for thumb movement and hand function, and arthritis here can cause significant pain, stiffness, and loss of dexterity. It is often linked to wear-and-tear processes, making it more common in older individuals or those with repetitive and constant hand use [73].

Epidemiology

CMC joint arthritis ranks among the most common forms of hand osteoarthritis, with a notably higher incidence in women. Approximately 25% of postmenopausal women are affected, whereas the condition is less common in men. Typically, the condition manifests in individuals over the age of 40, with its prevalence increasing with age. Various risk factors contribute to its development, including repetitive hand movements often seen in activities like writing, crafting, or manual labor. Obesity, which may exacerbate systemic inflammation, is another key factor. Additionally, a history of joint trauma or prior thumb injuries can heighten the likelihood of developing this form of arthritis [73, 74].

Clinical Presentation and Symptoms

Patients with CMC joint arthritis typically experience symptoms that significantly impair thumb and hand function. These may include pain at the base of the thumb, stiffness, reduced grip strength, and difficulty with activities requiring fine motor skills, such as buttoning a shirt or opening jars. Visible swelling and deformity of the joint may also be observed in more advanced cases [75, 76].

Pathophysiology

The pathophysiology of first carpometacarpal (CMC) arthritis involves the progressive degeneration of the articular cartilage within the trapeziometacarpal joint, leading to a cascade of structural and inflammatory changes. Repetitive motion and wear-and-tear gradually degrade the articular cartilage, resulting in the loss of its cushioning effect. This cartilage breakdown causes bone-on-bone contact, leading to pain and erosion of the joint surfaces [77].

Cartilage debris from the breakdown process triggers an inflammatory response in the synovial lining of the joint, known as synovitis. This inflammation is driven by cytokines such as interleukin-6 (IL-6) and tumor necrosis factor-alpha (TNF-α), which further exacerbate cartilage destruction and increase pain. In response to the damage, the body attempts to repair the joint, leading to the formation of bony outgrowths known as osteophytes. These osteophytes contribute to joint enlargement and deformity, further limiting function [77].

As the cartilage and ligament support deteriorate, the joint becomes unstable, resulting in subluxation or misalignment. Chronic inflammation also promotes increased vascular proliferation within the synovium, a process termed hypervascularity. This heightened vascular activity contributes to localized warmth and swelling, further compounding the symptoms of first CMC arthritis. Together, these processes create a cycle of degeneration, inflammation, and structural change that characterizes the condition [77].

Treatment Options

Treatment of CMC joint arthritis is managed by the severity of symptoms and functional impairment [73, 78–81]:

- *Non-Pharmacological.*
  - Changing activity routines to avoid repetitive strain
  - Use of supportive splints or braces (e.g., thumb spica splint) to stabilize the joint
  - Physical therapy to strengthen hand muscles and improve joint mechanics
- *Pharmacological*:
  - NSAIDs or acetaminophen for pain relief
  - Topical agents such as capsaicin or NSAID creams
  - Corticosteroid injections for severe inflammation and pain
- *Surgical* (for more advanced cases):
  - *Ligament Reconstruction and Tendon Interposition (LRTI)*: Removal of the trapezium bone and replacement with a tendon graft
  - *Joint Fusion (Arthrodesis)*: Fusing the bones to eliminate movement and pain
  - *Total Joint Arthroplasty*: Prosthetic joint replacement

- *Emerging Therapies*:
  - Platelet-rich plasma (PRP) or stem cell injections for regenerative effects
  - Biologics targeting inflammatory pathways

In conclusion, first CMC joint arthritis is a common and debilitating condition that significantly impacts hand function and quality of life. Early diagnosis and tailored interventions, including lifestyle adjustments, physical therapy, and advanced surgical options when needed, can greatly improve outcomes for affected individuals.

Dochu algorithm: carpometacarpal joint arthritis and first CMC	
External landmarks	1. Palpate the radial artery at the distal lower arm 2. Palpate the ulnar artery at the distal lower arm 3. Palpate the pulsating brachial artery at the level of the medial humeral epicondyle (in cases where the above 1 and 2 cannot be achieved)
Probe positioning	1. Transverse probe orientation at the carpal crease over the radial artery (Fig. 2.22) 2. Transverse probe orientation at the carpal crease over the ulnar artery (Fig. 2.23) 3. Transverse oblique probe orientation between the medial humeral epicondyle and the biceps brachii tendon (in cases where the above 1 and 2 cannot be achieved) (Fig. 2.24)
Target vessel	1. Radial artery (Figs. 2.25 and 2.26) 2. Ulnar artery (Figs. 2.27 and 2.28) 3. Brachial artery (Figs. 2.29 and 2.30)
Needle size	27G, length: 19 mm
Medication	Imipenem/Cilastatin (1 vial: 0.5 g/0.5 g) diluted with 10 cc of saline
Dosage	1 ml, 2 ml from the brachial artery
Cuff position	2–5th finger (optional)
Cuff compression duration	Deflate cuff 30 s after injection

*Depending on the patient's symptoms and distribution, Dochu is performed either on one artery or both. In cases where the puncturing of the radial and/or ulnar artery cannot be achieved, Dochu can be performed via the brachial artery

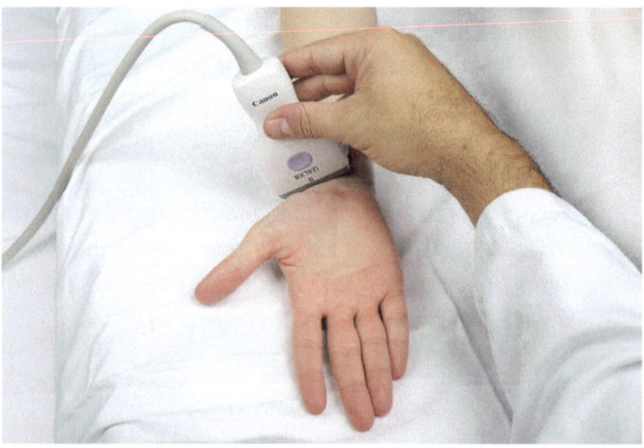

Fig. 2.22 Transverse probe orientation approx. 1 cm proximal to the carpal crease over the palpable radial artery

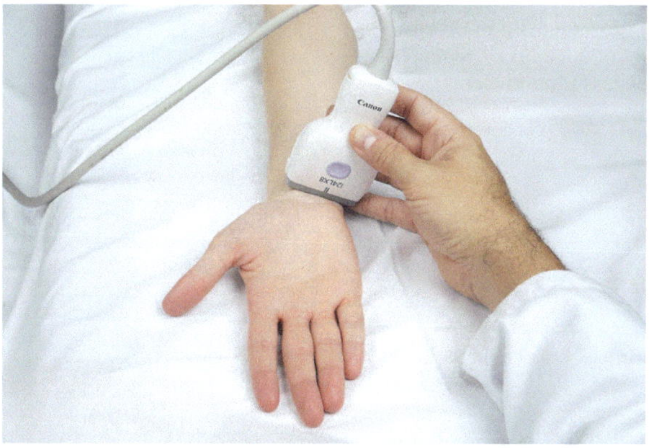

Fig. 2.23 Transverse probe orientation approx. 1 cm proximal to the carpal crease over the palpable ulnar artery

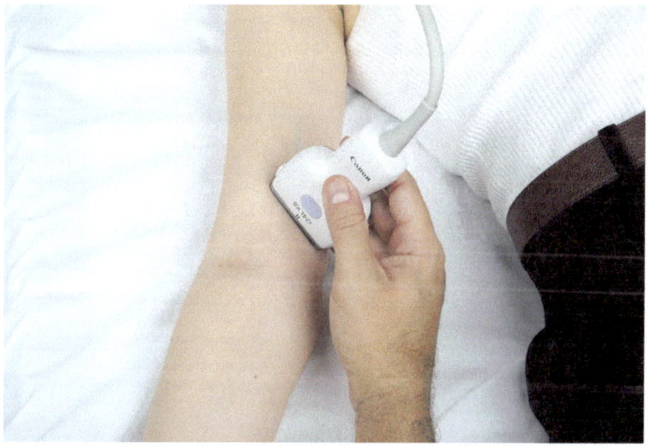

Fig. 2.24 Positioning of the probe between the palpable medial epicondyle and the medial distal biceps tendon in a transverse oblique orientation

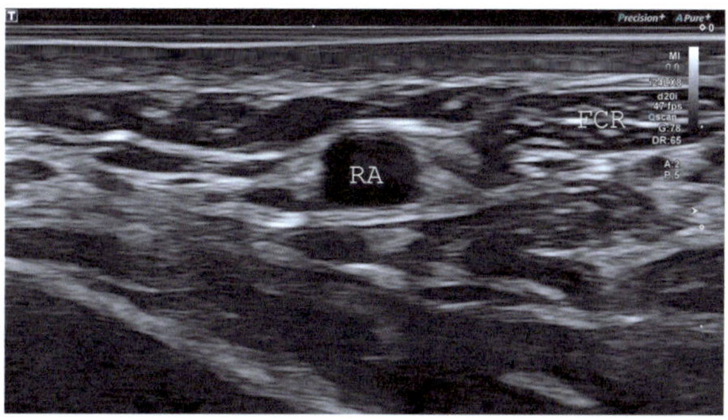

Fig. 2.25 Depiction of the radial artery (RA) at the level of the wrist radial to the flexor carpi radialis tendon (FCR)

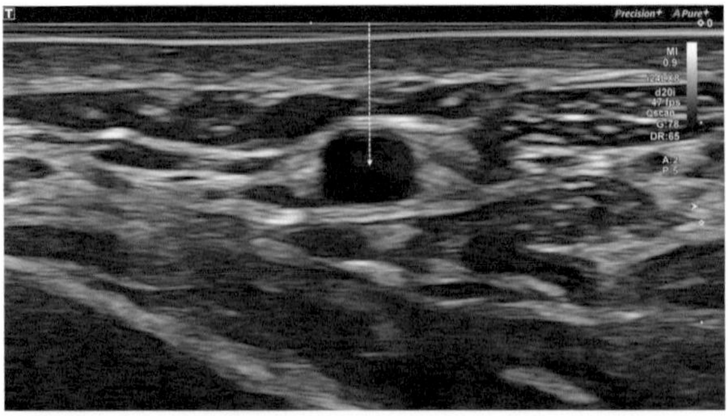

Fig. 2.26 Needle entry path in an out-of-plane access (dotted arrow)

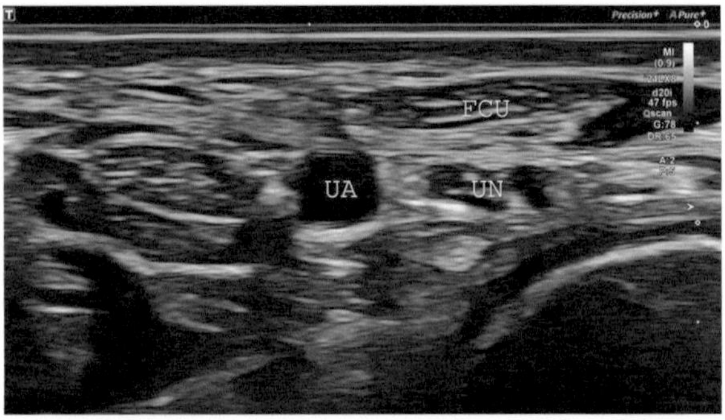

Fig. 2.27 Depiction of the ulnar artery (UA) radial to the ulnar nerve (UN) which is covered by the flecor carpi ulnaris tendon (FCU)

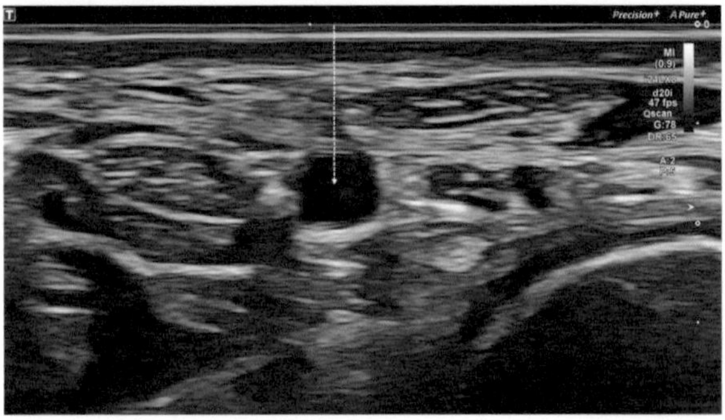

Fig. 2.28 Needle entry path in an out-of-plane access (dotted arrow). Cave: ulnar nerve!

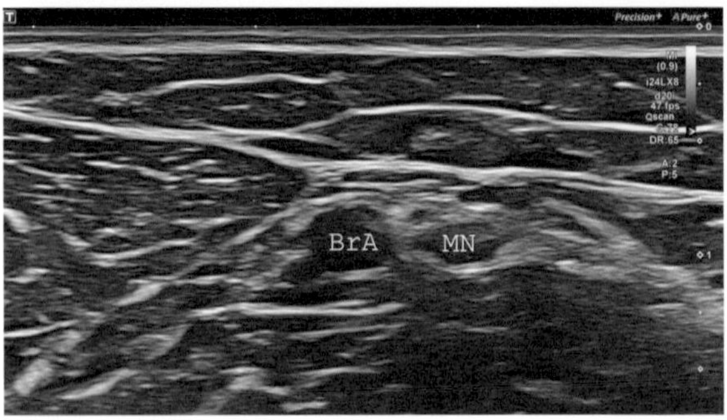

Fig. 2.29 Depiction of the brachial artery (BrA) mostly found immediately radial to the median nerve (MN)

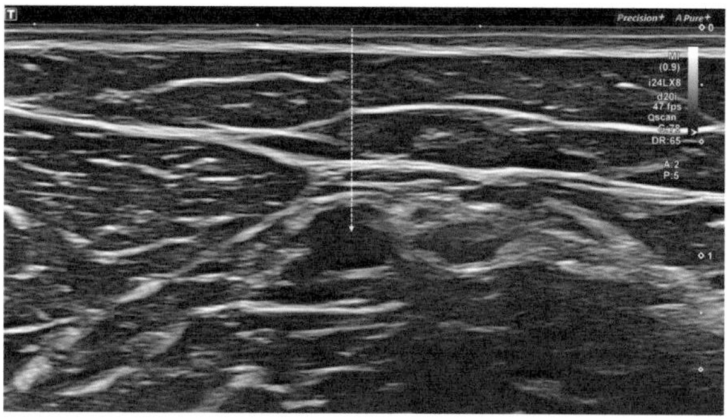

Fig. 2.30 Needle entry path in an out-of-plane access (dotted arrow). Cave: median nerve!

Heberden's Nodes

Introduction

Heberden's nodes are inflammations that develop on the distal interphalangeal (DIP) joints of the fingers and are a feature of osteoarthritis (OA), the most common form of arthritis [82]. Heberden's nodes predominantly affect the aging population, particularly women, and results in significant discomfort and functional impairment of the hand [83].

Epidemiology

From an epidemiological perspective, Heberden's nodes are a frequent manifestation of hand osteoarthritis, affecting up to 60% of individuals with the condition [83]. Its prevalence increases with age and particularly in women, who are disproportionately affected after the age of 50 [84]. Inherited predispositions linked to genes involving cartilage and joint stability have been identified as strong genetic components that eventually lead to the formation of Heberden's nodes [85]. While intrinsic contributors like genetics and aging play a key role in the manifestation of Heberden's nodes, external factors, including repetitive joint strain and chronic inflammation, also drive their development [86].

Clinical Presentation

The formation of Heberden's nodes is rooted in the mechanisms of osteoarthritis [87]. Intrinsically, aging diminishes the regenerative capacity of joint cartilage, making it more vulnerable to wear and tear [88]. In women, declining estrogen levels after menopause exacerbate cartilage fragility [89]. On the outside, repetitive mechanical stress from occupational or lifestyle activities, such as manual labor or typing, accelerates joint degeneration [90]. Over time, the cartilage erodes, and the body attempts to compensate by forming bony outgrowths, known as osteophytes, at the margins of the DIP joints. These outgrowths manifest as the often painful nodules characteristic of Heberden's nodes [85].

Patients with Heberden's nodes typically present with a distinct clinical profile. Visually, the nodes appear as inflammations on the DIP joints, often affecting both hands, although irregularity may occur [83]. Symptoms include pain that ranges from a blunt aches to sharp discomfort, particularly during activities involving finger use. Joint stiffness, particularly in the morning, is a common complaint but is usually short-lived [91]. Over time, patients may experience a reduced range of motion and visible joint deformities, which can significantly impact fine motor skills and grip strength. In the early stages, mild erythema or warmth may be noted over the nodes, indicating localized inflammation. Functionally, tasks requiring precision, such as buttoning clothes or holding utensils, become increasingly challenging [92].

Pathophysiology

The pathophysiology of Heberden's nodes involves a cascade of degenerative and reparative processes [93]. The condition begins with microtears in the articular cartilage, driven by mechanical stress and metabolic changes [94]. Enzymes like matrix metalloproteinases (MMPs) break down cartilage proteoglycans, leading to the loss of joint lubrication and smooth articulation. As the cartilage deteriorates, debris from its breakdown triggers localized inflammation in the synovium, although osteoarthritis is not primarily an inflammatory condition. IL-1 and TNF-α cytokines further exacerbate tissue damage and drive the process of osteophyte formation. Hypervascularity, characterized by increased blood vessel proliferation in the synovium and subchondral bone, contributes to inflammation and osteophyte growth, accounting for the occasional warmth and redness observed in affected joints. Over time, these processes culminate in the formation of the characteristic bony nodes [95].

Treatment Options

Management of Heberden's nodes focuses on alleviating symptoms, improving joint function, and slowing disease progression. Current treatment options include [96–103]:

- Non-pharmacological Treatments:
  - Lifestyle modifications, such as weight management to reduce joint stress and avoiding repetitive joint strain
  - Physical therapy involving range-of-motion exercises to maintain flexibility and strengthening exercises for hand and forearm muscles
  - Use of assistive devices, such as adaptive tools, to ease daily tasks

- Pharmacological Treatments:
  - Analgesics, including acetaminophen or NSAIDs, for pain relief
  - Topical treatments, such as capsaicin creams or NSAID gels, applied directly to the affected joints
  - Intra-articular injections of corticosteroids for severe pain and inflammation
- Procedural and Surgical Treatments:
  - Joint fusion (arthrodesis) for severe deformity and persistent pain unresponsive to conservative measures
  - Osteophyte removal for large osteophytes causing significant functional impairment
- Emerging Therapies:
  - Regenerative medicine approaches, such as platelet-rich plasma (PRP) injections, and stem cell therapy, which are being explored for their potential to repair cartilage damage
  - Biologics targeting inflammatory cytokines to modulate disease progression

In conclusion, Heberden's nodes are a defining feature of osteoarthritis, arising from a complex interplay of cartilage degradation, inflammation, and osteophyte formation. While the condition cannot be reversed, a combination of non-pharmacological, pharmacological, and surgical interventions can help manage symptoms and improve quality of life. Advances in regenerative medicine and biologic therapies hold promise for more effective treatments, offering hope for better outcomes in the future.

Dochu algorithm: Heberden's node	
External landmarks	1. Palpate the radial artery at the distal lower arm 2. Palpate the ulnar artery at the distal lower arm 3. Palpate the pulsating brachial artery at the level of the medial humeral epicondyle (in cases where the above 1 and 2 cannot be achieved)
Probe positioning	1. Transverse probe orientation at the carpal crease over the radial artery (Fig. 2.31) 2. Transverse probe orientation at the carpal crease over the ulnar artery (Fig. 2.32) 3. Transverse oblique probe orientation between the medial humeral epicondyle and the biceps brachii tendon (in cases where the above 1 and 2 cannot be achieved) (Fig. 2.33)
Target vessel	1. Radial artery (Figs. 2.34 and 2.35) 2. Ulnar artery (Figs. 2.36 and 2.37) 3. Brachial artery (Figs. 2.38 and 2.39)
Needle size	27G, length: 19 mm
Medication	Imipenem/Cilastatin (1vial: 0.5 g/0.5 g) diluted with 10 cc of saline
Dosage	1 ml each, 2 ml from the brachial artery
Cuff position	NA

*Depending on the patient's symptoms and distribution, Dochu is performed either on one artery or both. In cases where the puncturing of the radial and/or ulnar artery cannot be achieved, Dochu can be performed on the brachial artery

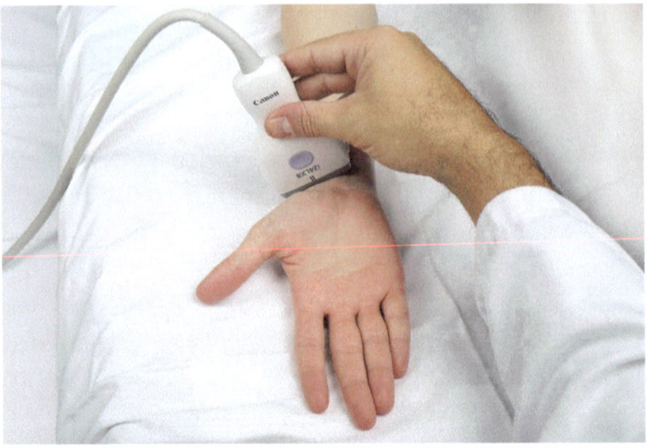

Fig. 2.31 Transverse probe orientation approx. 1 cm proximal to the carpal crease over the palpable radial artery

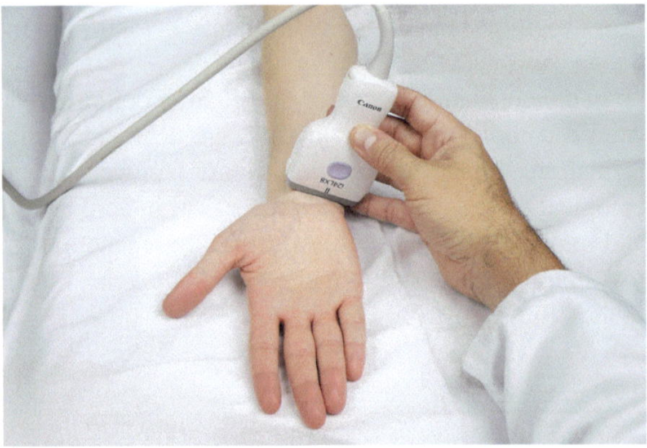

Fig. 2.32 Transverse probe orientation approx. 1 cm proximal to the carpal crease over the palpable ulnar artery

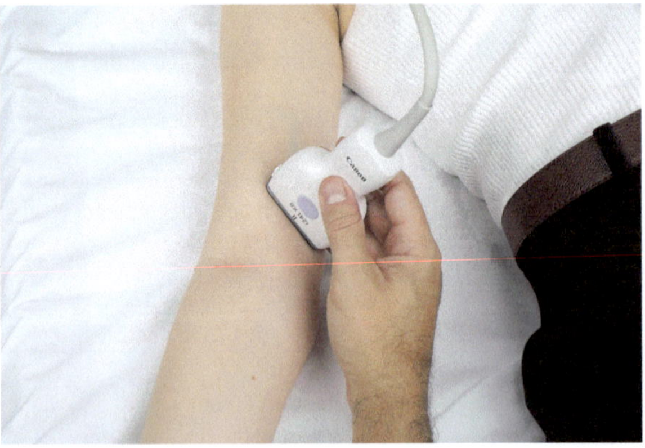

Fig. 2.33 Positioning of the probe between the palpable medial epicondyle and the medial distal biceps tendon in a transverse oblique orientation

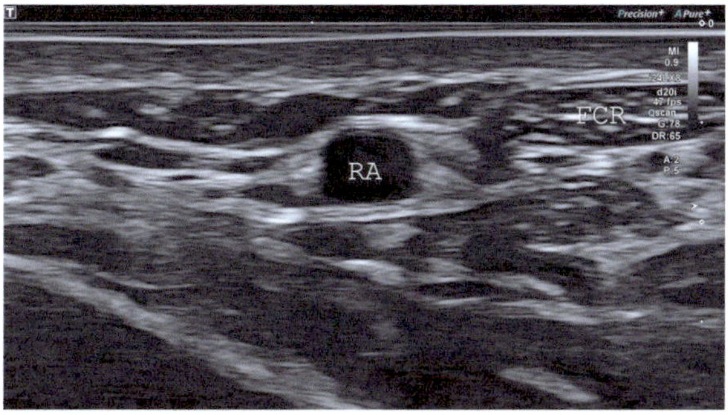

Fig. 2.34 Depiction of the radial artery (RA) at the level of the wrist radial to the flexor carpi radialis tendon (FCR)

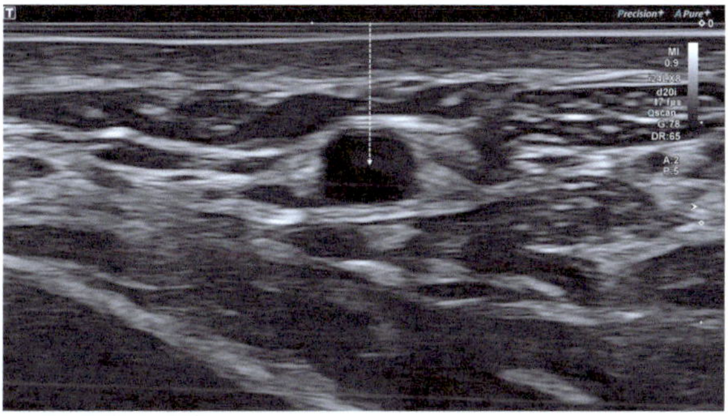

Fig. 2.35 Needle entry path in an out-of-plane access (dotted arrow)

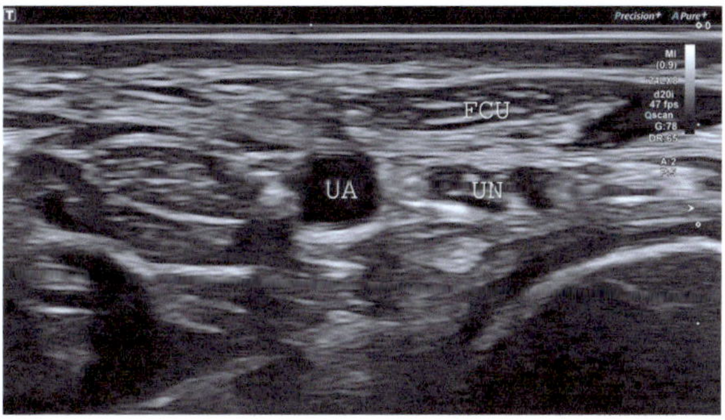

Fig. 2.36 Depiction of the ulnar artery (UA) radial to the ulnar nerve (UN) which is covered by the flexor carpi ulnaris tendon (FCU)

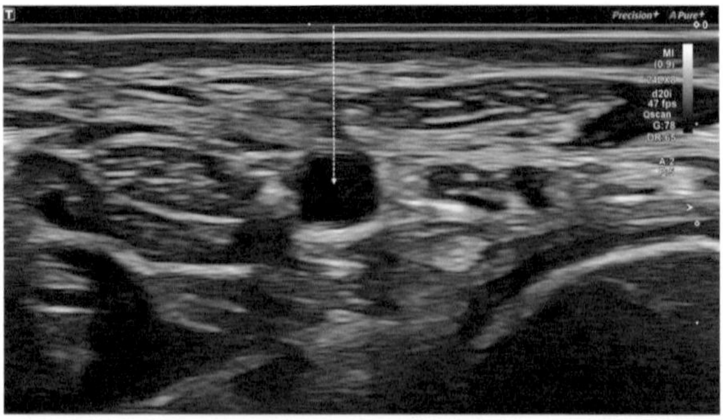

Fig. 2.37 Needle entry path in an out-of-plane access (dotted arrow). Cave: ulnar nerve!

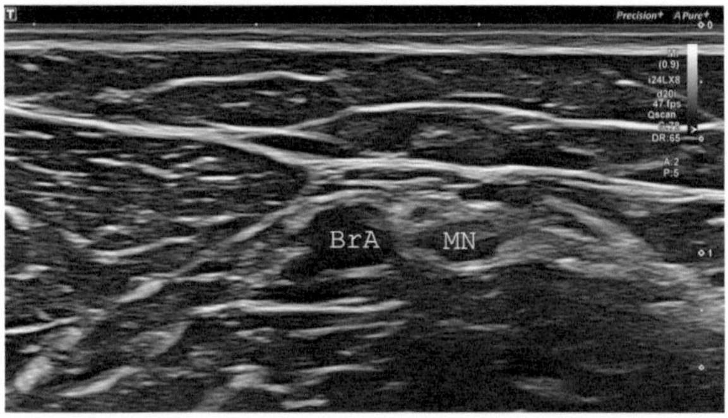

Fig. 2.38 Depiction of the brachial artery (BrA) mostly found immediately radial to the median nerve (MN)

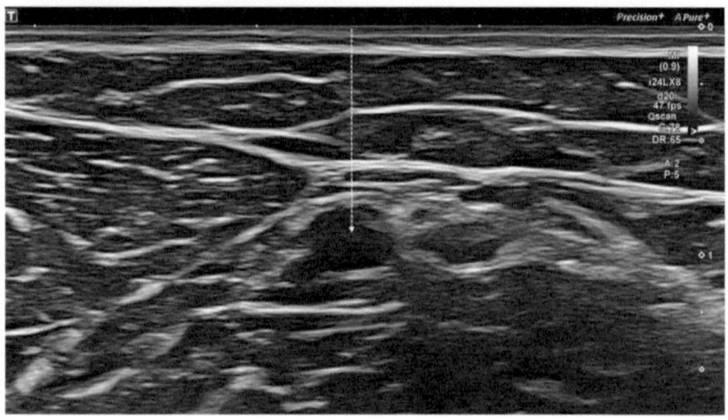

Fig. 2.39 Needle entry path in an out-of-plane access (dotted arrow). Cave: median nerve!

References

1. Brandt M, Sundstrup E, Jakobsen MD, Jay K, Colado JC, Wang Y, Zebis MK, Andersen LL. Association between neck/shoulder pain and trapezius muscle tenderness in office workers. Pain Res Treat. 2014;2014(1):352735.
2. Aarås A. Relationship between trapezius load and the incidence of musculoskeletal illness in the neck and shoulder. Int J Ind Ergon. 1994;14(4):341–8.
3. Cheung J, Kajaks T, Macdermid JC. The relationship between neck pain and physical activity. Open Orthop J J. 2013;7(4):521–9.

4. Cagnie B, Danneels L, Van Tiggelen D, De Loose V, Cambier D. Individual and work related risk factors for neck pain among office workers: a cross sectional study. Eur Spine J. 2007;16:679–86.
5. Shahidi B, Curran-Everett D, Maluf KS. Psychosocial, physical, and neurophysiological risk factors for chronic neck pain: a prospective inception cohort study. J Pain. 2015;16(12):1288–99.
6. Cohen SP, Hooten WM. Advances in the diagnosis and management of neck pain. BMJ. 2017;358:j3221.
7. Misailidou V, Malliou P, Beneka A, Karagiannidis A, Godolias G. Assessment of patients with neck pain: a review of definitions, selection criteria, and measurement tools. J Chiropr Med. 2010;9(2):49–59.
8. Takala EP. Pressure pain threshold on upper trapezius and levator scapulae muscles. Repeatability and relation to subjective symptoms in a working population. J Rehabil Med. 1990;22(2):63–8.
9. Visser B, van Dieën JH. Pathophysiology of upper extremity muscle disorders. J Electromyogr Kinesiol. 2006;16(1):1–16.
10. Hubbard DR. Chronic and recurrent muscle pain: pathophysiology and treatment, and review of pharmacologic studies. J Musculoskelet Pain. 1996;4(1–2):123–44.
11. Lee KJ, Han HY, Cheon SH, Park SH, Yong MS. The effect of forward head posture on muscle activity during neck protraction and retraction. J Phys Ther Sci. 2015;27(3):977–9.
12. Singla D, Veqar Z. Association between forward head, rounded shoulders, and increased thoracic kyphosis: a review of the literature. J Chiropr Med. 2017;16(3):220–9.
13. Gross A, Kay TM, Paquin JP, Blanchette S, Lalonde P, Christie T, Dupont G, Graham N, Burnie SJ, Gelley G, Goldsmith CH. Exercises for mechanical neck disorders. Cochrane Database Syst Rev. 2015;1(1):CD004250.
14. Sarig-Bahat H. Evidence for exercise therapy in mechanical neck disorders. Man Ther. 2003;8(1):10–20.
15. Park SH, Lee MM. Effects of lower trapezius strengthening exercises on pain, dysfunction, posture alignment, muscle thickness and contraction rate in patients with neck pain; randomized controlled trial. Med Sci Monit. 2020;26:e920208–1.
16. Nunes AMP, Moita JPAM. Effectiveness of physical and rehabilitation techniques in reducing pain in chronic trapezius myalgia: a systematic review and meta-analysis. Int J Osteopath Med. 2015;18(3):189–206
17. Bigliani LU, Perez-Sanz JR, Wolfe IN. Treatment of trapezius paralysis. J Bone Joint Surg Am. 1985;67(6):871–7.
18. Esenyel M, Caglar N, Aldemir T. Treatment of myofascial pain. Am J Phys Med Rehabil. 2000;79(1):48–52.
19. Thomas M, Bidwai A, Rangan A, Rees JL, Brownson P, Tennent D, Connor C, Kulkarni R. Glenohumeral osteoarthritis. Shoulder & Elbow. 2016;8(3):203–14.
20. Chillemi C, Franceschini V. Shoulder osteoarthritis. Arthritis. 2013;2013(1):370231.
21. Ibounig T, Simons T, Launonen A, Paavola M. Glenohumeral osteoarthritis: an overview of etiology and diagnostics. Scand J Surg. 2021;110(3):441–51.
22. Crane C, Wagner C, Wong S, Hall B, Hull J, Irwin K, Williams K, Brooks A. Glenohumeral osteoarthritis: a biological advantage or a missed diagnosis? J Clin Med. 2024;13(8):2341.
23. Escamilla RF, Hooks TR, Wilk KE. Optimal management of shoulder impingement syndrome. Open Access J Sports Med. 2014;5:13–24.
24. Koester MC, George MS, Kuhn JE. Shoulder impingement syndrome. Am J Med. 2005;118(5):452–5.
25. Ansok CB, Muh SJ. Optimal management of glenohumeral osteoarthritis. Orthop Res Rev. 2018;Volume 10:9–18.
26. Yamamoto N, Szymski D, Voss A, Ishikawa H, Muraki T, Cunha RA, Ejnisman B, Noack J, McCarty E, Mulcahey MK, Itoi E. Non-operative management of shoulder osteoarthritis: current concepts. J ISAKOS. 2023;8(5):289–95.

27. Yao Y, Xie W, Opoku M, Vithran DTA, Li Z, Li Y. Cryotherapy and thermotherapy in the management of osteoarthritis and rheumatoid arthritis: a comprehensive review. Fundam Res. 2024;5(6):2409–31.
28. Gellman H. Tennis elbow (lateral epicondylitis). Orthop Clin North Am. 1992;23(1):75–82.
29. Tosti R, Jennings J, Sewards JM. Lateral epicondylitis of the elbow. Am J Med. 2013;126(4):357–e1.
30. Buchanan BK, Varacallo M. Tennis elbow (lateral epicondylitis). StatPearls [Internet]; 2019.
31. McMurtrie A, Watts AC. (vi) Tennis elbow and Golfer's elbow. Orthop Trauma. 2012;26(5):337–44.
32. Kiel J, Kaiser K. Golfers elbow. In: StatPearls [internet]. StatPearls Publishing; 2023.
33. Cutts S, Gangoo S, Modi N, Pasapula C. Tennis elbow: a clinical review article. J Orthop. 2020;17:203–7.
34. Keijsers R, de Vos RJ, Kuijer PPF, van den Bekerom MP, van der Woude HJ, Eygendaal D. Tennis elbow. Shoulder & Elbow. 2019;11(5):384–92.
35. Walker-Bone K, Palmer KT, Reading I, Coggon D, Cooper C. Occupation and epicondylitis: a population-based study. Rheumatology. 2012;51(2):305–10.
36. Konarski W, Poboży T, Kotela A, Hordowicz M, Poboży K. Ultrasound in the differential diagnosis of medial epicondylalgia and medial elbow pain—imaging findings and narrative literature review. Healthcare. 2022;10(8):1529. MDPI
37. Taylor SA, Hannafin JA. Evaluation and management of elbow tendinopathy. Sports Health. 2012;4(5):384–93.
38. Walz DM, Newman JS, Konin GP, Ross G. Epicondylitis: pathogenesis, imaging, and treatment. Radiographics. 2010;30(1):167–84.
39. Orchard J, Kountouris A. The management of tennis elbow. BMJ. 2011:342.
40. Struijs PA, Smidt N, Arola H, Van Dijk CN, Buchbinder R, Assendelft WJ, Cochrane Musculoskeletal Group. Orthotic devices for the treatment of tennis elbow. Cochrane Database Syst Rev. 1996:2010(1).
41. Kamien M. A rational management of tennis elbow. Sports Med. 1990;9:173–91.
42. Tyler TF, Nicholas SJ, Schmitt BM, Mullaney M, Hogan DE. Clinical outcomes of the addition of eccentrics for rehabilitation of previously failed treatments of golfers elbow. Int J Sports Phys Ther. 2014;9(3):365.
43. Ciccotti MC, Schwartz MA, Ciccotti MG. Diagnosis and treatment of medial epicondylitis of the elbow. Clin Sports Med. 2004;23(4):693–705.
44. Fakoya AO, Tarzian M, Sabater EL, Burgos DM, Marty GIM. de Quervain's disease: a discourse on etiology, diagnosis, and treatment. Cureus. 2023;15(4):e38079.
45. Rutkowski M, Rutkowski K. Potential effects, diagnosis, and management of De Quervain Tenosynovitis in the aesthetics community: a brief review, case example, and illustrative exercises. J Clin Aesthet Dermatol. 2023;16(9 Suppl 2):S28.
46. Wolf JM, Sturdivant RX, Owens BD. Incidence of de Quervain's tenosynovitis in a young, active population. J Hand Surg Am. 2009;34(1):112–5.
47. Hassan K, Sohn A, Shi L, Lee M, Wolf JM. De Quervain tenosynovitis: an evaluation of the epidemiology and utility of multiple injections using a national database. J Hand Surg Am. 2022;47(3):284–e1.
48. Keidan T, Saleh S, Gannot G, Oron A. De Quervain's tenosynovitis-clinical presentation and treatment. Harefuah. 2022;161(11):706–8.
49. Ilyas AM, Ast M, Schaffer AA, Thoder J. De quervain tenosynovitis of the wrist. JAAOS. 2007;15(12):757–64.
50. Goel R, Abzug JM. de Quervain's tenosynovitis: a review of the rehabilitative options. Hand. 2015;10(1):1–5.
51. Challoumas D, Ramasubbu R, Rooney E, Seymour-Jackson E, Putti A, Millar NL. Management of de Quervain tenosynovitis: a systematic review and network meta-analysis. JAMA Netw Open. 2023;6(10):e2337001.
52. Ippolito JA, Hauser S, Patel J, Vosbikian M, Ahmed I. Nonsurgical treatment of De Quervain tenosynovitis: a prospective randomized trial. Hand. 2020;15(2):215–9.

53. Allbrook V. 'The side of my wrist hurts':'De Quervain's tenosynovitis. Aust J Gen Pract. 2019;48(11):753–6.
54. Ilyas AM. Nonsurgical treatment for de Quervain's tenosynovitis. J Hand Surg. 2009;34(5):928–9.
55. Guo Q, Wang Y, Xu D, Nossent J, Pavlos NJ, Xu J. Rheumatoid arthritis: pathological mechanisms and modern pharmacologic therapies. Bone research. 2018;6(1):15.
56. Radu AF, Bungau SG. Management of rheumatoid arthritis: an overview. Cells. 2021;10(11):2857.
57. Firestein GS. Evolving concepts of rheumatoid arthritis. Nature. 2003;423(6937):356–61.
58. Venetsanopoulou AI, Alamanos Y, Voulgari PV, Drosos AA. Epidemiology and risk factors for rheumatoid arthritis development. Mediterr J Rheumatol. 2023;34(4):404.
59. Chancay MG, Guendsechadze SN, Blanco I. Types of pain and their psychosocial impact in women with rheumatoid arthritis. Women's Midlife Health. 2019;5:1–9.
60. Gabriel SE. The epidemiology of rheumatoid arthritis. Rheum Dis Clin North Am. 2001;27(2):269–81.
61. Grassi W, De Angelis R, Lamanna G, Cervini C. The clinical features of rheumatoid arthritis. Eur J Radiol. 1998;27:S18–24.
62. Ragan C, Farrington E. The clinical features of rheumatoid arthritis: prognostic indices. JAMA. 1962;181(8):663–7.
63. Mohammed RH, Bansal P. Hand and wrist rheumatoid arthritis. StatPearls [online]; 2021.
64. Jutley GS, Latif ZP, Raza K. Symptoms in individuals at risk of rheumatoid arthritis. Best Pract Res Clin Rheumatol. 2017;31(1):59–70.
65. Volkov M, van Schie KA, van der Woude D. Autoantibodies and B cells: the ABC of rheumatoid arthritis pathophysiology. Immunol Rev. 2020;294(1):148–63.
66. Jang S, Kwon EJ, Lee JJ. Rheumatoid arthritis: pathogenic roles of diverse immune cells. Int J Mol Sci. 2022;23(2):905.
67. Li K, Wang M, Zhao L, Liu Y, Zhang X. ACPA-negative rheumatoid arthritis: from immune mechanisms to clinical translation. EBioMedicine. 2022;83:*104233*.
68. Kavuncu V, Evcik D. Physiotherapy in rheumatoid arthritis. Medscape Gen Med. 2004;6(2):3.
69. Almeida PHTQD, Pontes TB, Matheus JPC, Muniz LF, Mota LMHD. Occupational therapy in rheumatoid arthritis: what rheumatologists need to know? Rev Bras Reumatol. 2015;55:272–80.
70. Burmester GR, Pope JE. Novel treatment strategies in rheumatoid arthritis. Lancet. 2017;389(10086):2338–48.
71. Bullock J, Rizvi SA, Saleh AM, Ahmed SS, Do DP, Ansari RA, Ahmed J. Rheumatoid arthritis: a brief overview of the treatment. Med Princ Pract. 2019;27(6):501–7.
72. Smolen JS, Aletaha D, Koeller M, Weisman MH, Emery P. New therapies for treatment of rheumatoid arthritis. Lancet. 2007;370(9602):1861–74.
73. Gillis J, Calder K, Williams J. Review of thumb carpometacarpal arthritis classification, treatment and outcomes. Can Jo Plastic Surg. 2011;19(4):134–8.
74. Haugen IK, Englund M, Aliabadi P, Niu J, Clancy M, Kvien TK, Felson DT. Prevalence, incidence and progression of hand osteoarthritis in the general population: the Framingham osteoarthritis study. Ann Rheum Dis. 2011;70(9):1581–6.
75. Dias R, Chandrasenan J, Rajaratnam V, Burke FD. Basal thumb arthritis. Postgrad Med J. 2007;83(975):40–3.
76. Van Heest AE, Kallemeier P. Thumb carpal metacarpal arthritis. JAAOS. 2008;16(3):140–51.
77. Pellegrini VD Jr. Osteoarthritis of the trapeziometacarpal joint: the pathophysiology of articular cartilage degeneration. I. Anatomy and pathology of the aging joint. J Hand Surg Am. 1991;16(6):967–74.
78. Yuan F, Aliu O, Chung KC, Mahmoudi E. Evidence-based practice in the surgical treatment of thumb carpometacarpal joint arthritis. J Hand Surg Am. 2017;42(2):104–12.
79. Baker RH, Al-Shukri J, Davis TR. Evidence-based medicine: thumb basal joint arthritis. Plast Reconstr Surg. 2017;139(1):256e–66e.

80. Hamasaki T, Lalonde L, Harris P, Bureau NJ, Gaudreault N, Ziegler D, Choiniere M. Efficacy of treatments and pain management for trapeziometacarpal (thumb base) osteoarthritis: protocol for a systematic review. BMJ Open. 2015;5(10):e008904.
81. Higgenbotham C, Boyd A, Busch M, Heaton D, Trumble T. Optimal management of thumb basal joint arthritis: challenges and solutions. Orthop Res Rev. 2017;9:93–9.
82. Urbano FL. Heberden's nodes. Hosp Physician. 2001;38:29–31.
83. Duruöz MT, Gürsoy DE, Tuncer T, Altan L, Ayhan F, Bal A, Bilgilisoy M, Cerrahoğlu L, Çapkın E, Çay HF, Çevik R. The clinical, functional, and radiological features of hand osteoarthritis: TLAR-osteoarthritis multi-center cohort study. Arch Rheumatol. 2022;37(3):375.
84. Kalichman L, Hernández-Molina G. Hand osteoarthritis: an epidemiological perspective. Semin Arthritis Rheum. 2010;39(6):465–76. WB Saunders.
85. Brandi ML, Gennari L, Cerinic MM, Becherini L, Falchetti A, Masi L, Gennari C, Reginster JY. Genetic markers of osteoarticular disorders: facts and hopes. Arthritis Res Ther. 2001;3:1–11.
86. Li X, Li C, Zhang W, Wang Y, Qian P, Huang H. Inflammation and aging: signaling pathways and intervention therapies. Signal Transduct Target Ther. 2023;8(1):239.
87. Hoaglund FT. Clinical manifestations of osteoarthrosis. Clin Rheum Dis. 1976;2(3):543–56.
88. Li Y, Wei X, Zhou J, Wei L. The age-related changes in cartilage and osteoarthritis. Biomed Res Int. 2013;2013(1):916530.
89. Lou C, Xiang G, Weng Q, Chen Z, Chen D, Wang Q, Zhang D, Zhou B, He D, Chen H. Menopause is associated with articular cartilage degeneration: a clinical study of knee joint in 860 women. Menopause. 2016;23(11):1239–46.
90. Buckwalter JA, Anderson DD, Brown TD, Tochigi Y, Martin JA. The roles of mechanical stresses in the pathogenesis of osteoarthritis: implications for treatment of joint injuries. Cartilage. 2013;4(4):286–94.
91. WebMD. Heberden's Nodes: symptoms, causes, and treatments. 2024. [online] Available at: https://www.webmd.com/osteoarthritis/heberdens-nodes-symptoms-causes-treatments [Access date: 3 December 2024].
92. Ceceli E, Gül S, Borman PN, Uysal SR, Okumuş M. Hand function in female patients with hand osteoarthritis: relation with radiological progression. Hand. 2012;7(3):335–40.
93. Thaper A, Zhang W, Wright G, Doherty M. Relationship between Heberden's nodes and underlying radiographic changes of osteoarthritis. Ann Rheum Dis. 2005;64(8):1214–6.
94. Man GS, Mologhianu G. Osteoarthritis pathogenesis–a complex process that involves the entire joint. J Med Life. 2014;7(1):37.
95. Mukherjee A, Das B. The role of inflammatory mediators and matrix metalloproteinases (MMPs) in the progression of osteoarthritis. Biomater Biosyst. 2024;13:100090.
96. Sofat N, Kuttapitiya A. Future directions for the management of pain in osteoarthritis. Int J Clin Rheumtol. 2014;9(2):197.
97. Arthritis Foundation. Treatments for osteoarthritis. 2022. [online] Available at: https://www.arthritis.org/health-wellness/treatment/treatment-plan/disease-management/treatments-for-osteoarthritis [Accessed 3 Dec. 2024].
98. Mayo Clinic. Osteoarthritis - Diagnosis & treatment. 2021. [online] Available at: https://www.mayoclinic.org/diseases-conditions/osteoarthritis/diagnosis-treatment/drc-20351930 [Access date: 3 December 2024].
99. Arthritis Foundation. Hand surgery for arthritis. n.d. [online] Available at: https://www.arthritis.org/health-wellness/treatment/joint-surgery/preplanning/hand-surgery-for-arthritis [Access date: 3 December 2024].
100. Arthritis Foundation. Using ring splints to support finger joints. n.d. [online] Available at: https://www.arthritis.org/health-wellness/healthy-living/managing-pain/joint-protection/using-ring-splints-to-support-finger-joints [Access date: 3 December 2024].

101. Mayo Clinic. Hand exercises for people with arthritis. 2023. [online] Available at: https://www.mayoclinic.org/diseases-conditions/arthritis/in-depth/arthritis/art-20546847 [Access date: 3 December 2024].
102. Arthritis Foundation. Injections for arthritis in hands. n.d. [online] Available at: https://www.arthritis.org/health-wellness/healthy-living/managing-pain/pain-relief-solutions/hand-injections [Access date: 3 December 2024].
103. Arthritis Foundation. Treatment guidelines for osteoarthritis. n.d. [online] Available at: https://www.arthritis.org/diseases/more-about/guidelines-for-osteoarthritis-treatments [Access date: 3 December 2024].

Lower Extremity

3

Trochanteric Bursitis

Introduction

Trochanteric bursitis, also known as greater trochanteric pain syndrome (GTPS), is an inflammatory condition affecting the bursa located over the greater trochanter of the femur. The bursa functions as a cushion, reducing friction between the iliotibial band, gluteal tendons, and the greater trochanter. This condition is a common cause of lateral hip pain and is often associated with overuse, trauma, or degenerative changes in the surrounding tendons [1–3].

Epidemiology

Trochanteric bursitis is prevalent in both active and sedentary populations, particularly among middle-aged and older adults. It affects up to 15% of adults, with higher rates observed in women, and is frequently seen in runners, athletes, or individuals involved in repetitive hip movements. The condition is most common in individuals aged 40 to 60 years, with women being more affected, possibly due to differences in pelvic biomechanics. Risk factors include overuse or repetitive hip movements, such as running or walking on uneven surfaces, obesity or sudden weight gain, leg length discrepancies or altered gait mechanics, and previous hip surgeries, including total hip replacements. Underlying conditions like osteoarthritis or rheumatoid arthritis also increase the risk [1, 4, 5].

Y. Okuno et al., *Ultrasound-guided Musculoskeletal Embolotherapies using the "Dochu" Technique*, https://doi.org/10.1007/978-3-032-17250-1_3

Clinical Presentation and Symptoms

Patients with trochanteric bursitis often experience localized lateral hip pain, which is most pronounced over the greater trochanter. The pain typically worsens with activities such as walking, climbing stairs, or lying on the affected side. Initially sharp during movement, the pain may transition to a dull ache. Tenderness over the greater trochanter is a common finding upon palpation, and some patients may exhibit mild localized swelling in the lateral hip region. Stiffness or tightness in the hip and surrounding muscles is often reported, particularly after prolonged sitting or inactivity. Functional limitations include difficulty performing activities involving hip movement, such as getting out of a car or standing from a seated position. Discomfort when lying on the affected side can disrupt sleep [1, 6–8].

Pathophysiology

Trochanteric bursitis develops as a result of inflammation and biomechanical strain on the bursa and surrounding structures. Mechanical overload from repeated friction or trauma caused by the iliotibial band and gluteal tendons rubbing over the greater trochanter irritates the bursa. This irritation leads to inflammation, causing swelling, pain, and tenderness. Chronic inflammation or overuse can result in tendinopathy of the gluteus medius and minimus tendons. Hypervascularity, or increased blood vessel formation in the bursa, contributes to persistent inflammation and discomfort. Gait abnormalities or structural differences place additional stress on the hip, perpetuating the condition [9–11].

Treatment Options

Management focuses on alleviating pain, reducing inflammation, and addressing underlying biomechanical issues [1, 5, 12–14]:

- *Non-Pharmacological*:
  - *Rest and Activity Modification*:
    Avoid activities that exacerbate symptoms, such of trochanteric bursitis as running or prolonged standing
  - *Physical Therapy*:
    Strengthening exercises for the gluteal and hip abductors to improve stability
    Stretching exercises for the iliotibial band and hip flexors
    Gait retraining and balance exercises to correct biomechanics
  - *Ice or Heat Therapy*:
    Ice for acute pain and inflammation; heat for muscle tightness

  - *Assistive Devices*:
    Use of a cane or walker to reduce weight-bearing stress on the affected hip
- *Pharmacological*:
  - NSAIDs for pain relief and inflammation control
  - Topical analgesics for localized pain management
  - Corticosteroid injections into the bursa for persistent or severe symptoms
- *Procedural/Surgical*:
  - *Aspiration*:
    Removal of excess fluid from the bursa to reduce swelling and pain
  - *Surgical Bursectomy*:
    Removal of the inflamed bursa in refractory cases
  - *Tendon Repair or Release*:
    Repairing or releasing the gluteal tendons if tendinopathy is present
- *Emerging Therapies*:
  - Platelet-rich plasma (PRP) injections to promote tendon and bursa healing
  - Ultrasound-guided therapies for precision treatment of the inflamed bursa
  - Stem cell therapy for regenerative healing in chronic cases

In conclusion, trochanteric bursitis is a common condition that significantly impacts mobility and quality of life. Early recognition and treatment, including activity modification, physical therapy, and anti-inflammatory measures, can effectively manage symptoms and prevent progression. Advanced therapies and surgical options provide relief for refractory cases, restoring function and comfort to affected individuals.

Dochu algorithm: trochanteric bursitis	
External landmarks	Palpation of the pulsating common femoral artery
Probe positioning	Transverse probe orientation over the common femoral artery depicting the femoral bifurcation (Figs. 3.1 and 3.2)
Target vessel	1. Deep femoral artery (Figs. 3.3 and 3.4) 2. Common femoral artery if the deep femoral artery cannot be reached (Figs. 3.5 and 3.6)
Needle size	27G, length: 25–38 mm
Medication	Imipenem/Cilastatin (1 vial: 0.5 g/0.5 g) diluted with 10 cc of saline
Dosage	4 ml
Cuff position	Femoral region (Note: A standard upper-arm blood pressure cuff is too small for effective compression; use a larger thigh cuff!)
Cuff compression duration	Deflate cuff 30 s after injection

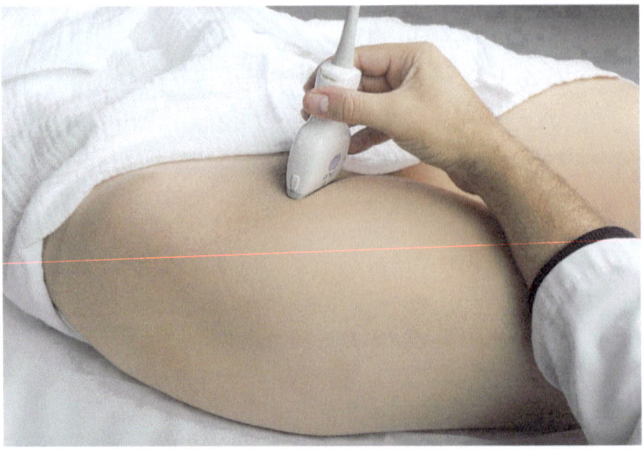

Fig. 3.1 Transverse probe orientation slightly distal to the palpable common femoral artery at the level of the femoral bifurcation

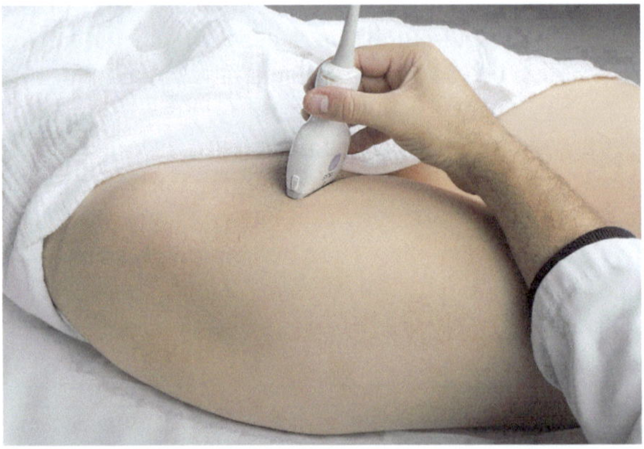

Fig. 3.2 Transverse probe orientation over the palpable common femoral artery

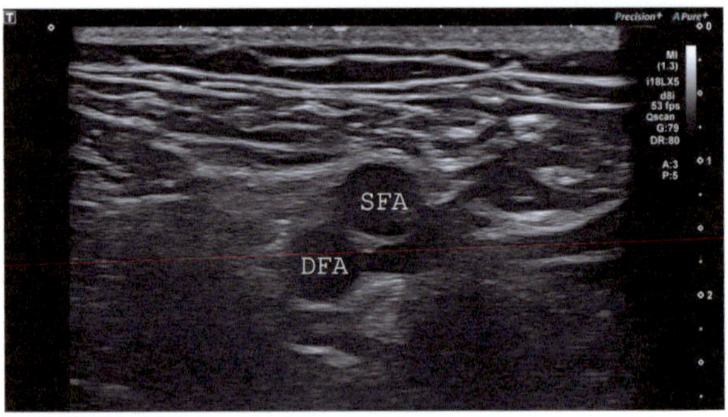

Fig. 3.3 Femoral bifurcation with depiction of the superficial femoral artery (SFA) and deep femoral artery (DFA)

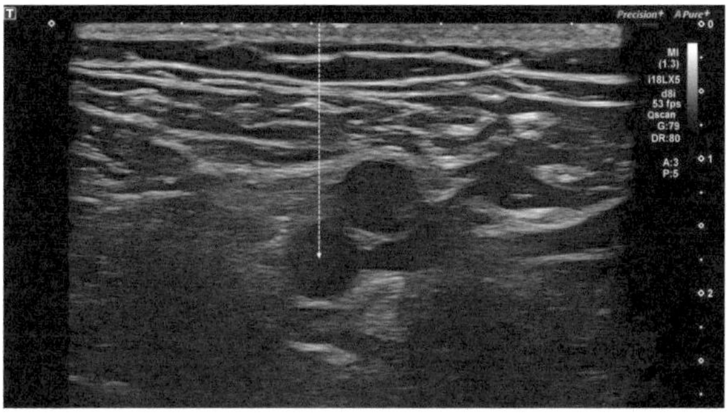

Fig. 3.4 Needle entry path in an out-of-plane access (dotted arrow) immediately lateral to the superficial femoral artery

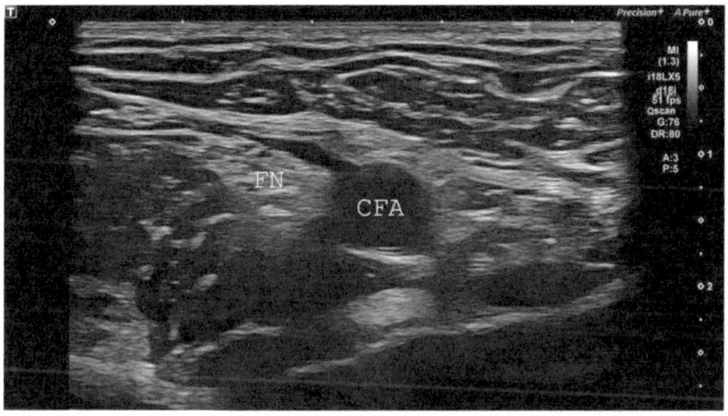

Fig. 3.5 Depiction of the common femoral artery (CFA) distal to the inguinal ligament and medial to the femoral nerve (FN)

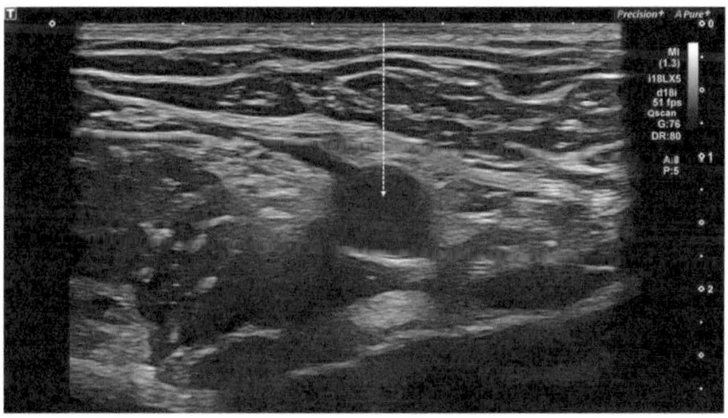

Fig. 3.6 Needle entry path in an out-of-plane access (dotted arrow). Cave: femoral nerve

Knee Osteoarthritis (OA)

Introduction

Knee osteoarthritis (OA) is a degenerative joint disease characterized by the progressive breakdown of cartilage, changes in subchondral bone, and synovial inflammation. It is one of the leading causes of pain and disability worldwide, severely impacting mobility and quality of life. The condition is commonly associated with aging, obesity, joint injuries, and repetitive stress on the knee [15].

Epidemiology

Knee OA is a widespread condition affecting millions of people globally and is more prevalent in certain populations. Approximately 10–15% of individuals over the age of 60 are affected, and the lifetime risk of developing symptomatic knee OA is estimated to be 45%. The incidence of knee OA increases with age, particularly after 50, and women are more likely to develop the condition, especially following menopause. Obesity is a significant risk factor, as excess weight increases joint loading and systemic inflammation. Previous joint injuries, such as trauma or surgeries like ACL repair, also elevate the risk of developing OA. Additionally, repetitive stress from occupational or recreational activities involving knee strain contributes to its onset [16–18].

Clinical Presentation and Symptoms

Patients with knee OA often experience a range of symptoms and functional limitations. Pain is typically described as a deep, aching sensation in the knee, which worsens with activity, such as prolonged standing, walking, or climbing stairs. In advanced stages, pain may persist even at rest or during the night. Stiffness is another common symptom, with morning stiffness usually lasting less than 30 min and stiffness occurring after prolonged inactivity, known as the "gelling phenomenon." [19, 20]

Intermittent swelling due to synovial inflammation or joint effusion is frequently reported, alongside crepitus, a grinding or cracking sensation during knee movement. Reduced range of motion often leads to difficulty in bending or straightening the knee, while deformities such as bow-leg (varus) or knock-knee (valgus) alignment may develop in severe cases. Functional limitations, such as difficulty squatting, kneeling, or rising from a chair, are common and significantly affect daily life [19, 21].

Pathophysiology

The progression of knee OA involves a combination of mechanical and biochemical processes. Repeated stress on the knee joint leads to the degradation of articular cartilage, resulting in the loss of cushioning and increased joint friction. As cartilage wears away, the underlying subchondral bone becomes exposed, triggering sclerosis and the formation of osteophytes, or bone spurs.

Synovial inflammation, or synovitis, occurs when synovial cells respond to cartilage debris and inflammatory mediators such as interleukin-1 (IL-1) and tumor necrosis factor-alpha (TNF-α). Hypervascularity in the synovium contributes to joint warmth and swelling during inflammation. Progressive cartilage loss results in joint space narrowing, leading to mechanical instability. Muscle weakness, particularly in the quadriceps, exacerbates joint instability and accelerates cartilage degradation [22].

Treatment Options

Management of knee OA is focused on pain relief, improving function, and slowing disease progression [23–27]:

- *Non-Pharmacological*:
  - *Weight Loss*: Reduces joint load and systemic inflammation
  - *Physical Therapy*:
    Strengthening exercises for quadriceps and hamstrings
    Range-of-motion and flexibility exercises
  - *Assistive Devices*:
    Braces or orthotics for joint stability
    Canes or walkers to reduce joint loading
  - *Lifestyle Modifications*:
    Avoiding activities that exacerbate symptoms
    Low-impact exercises like swimming or cycling
- *Pharmacological*:
  - NSAIDs for pain and inflammation
  - Acetaminophen for mild pain relief
  - Topical agents like capsaicin or diclofenac gel
  - Intra-articular corticosteroid injections for acute symptom flares
  - Viscosupplementation with hyaluronic acid for lubrication and pain relief
- *Procedural/Surgical*:
  - Arthroscopic debridement for mild cases with mechanical symptoms
  - Osteotomy to correct alignment in younger patients
  - Partial or total knee replacement in advanced cases with severe pain and functional limitation
- *Emerging Therapies*:
  - Platelet-rich plasma (PRP) injections to promote cartilage repair
  - Stem cell therapy for cartilage regeneration
  - Biologic agents targeting inflammatory mediators (e.g., IL-1 inhibitors)

In conclusion, knee OA is a significant public health issue due to its prevalence and impact on mobility. Early diagnosis, lifestyle modifications, and structured rehabilitation programs can slow disease progression and enhance quality of life. Advances in regenerative medicine and surgical techniques offer hope for more effective long-term solutions for severe cases.

Dochu algorithm: knee osteoarthritis	
External landmarks	Palpation of the pulsating popliteal artery in the popliteal fossa
Probe positioning	Transverse probe orientation over the popliteal artery with a medial-oblique needle entry (Fig. 3.7)
Target vessel	Popliteal artery (Figs. 3.8 and 3.9)
Needle size	25G, length: 38–62 mm
Medication	Imipenem/Cilastatin (1 vial: 0.5 g/0.5 g) diluted with 10 cc of saline
Dosage	5–10 ml
Cuff position	Lower leg
Cuff compression duration	Deflate cuff 30 s after injection

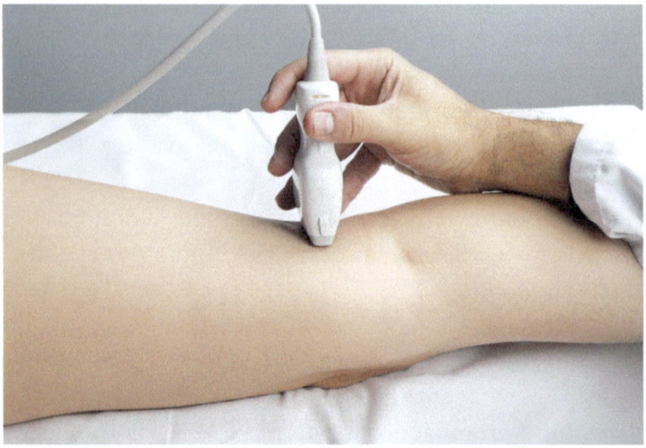

Fig. 3.7 Transverse probe orientation over the palpable popliteal artery approx. 3 cm proximal to the fibular head

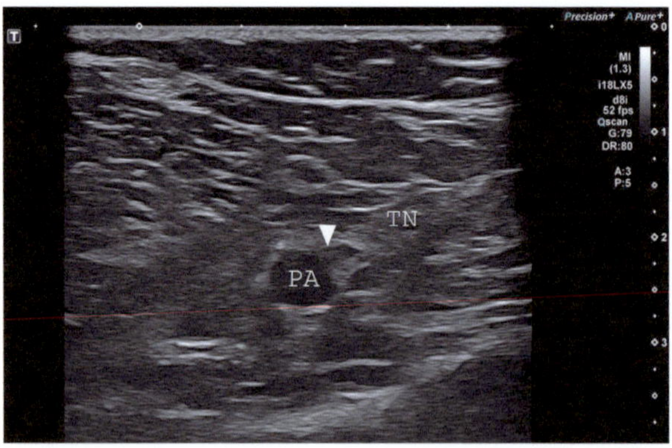

Fig. 3.8 Using compression, the popliteal artery (PA) can be depicted at the level of the popliteal fossa. Compressed popliteal vein (arrowhead). Tibial nerve (TN)

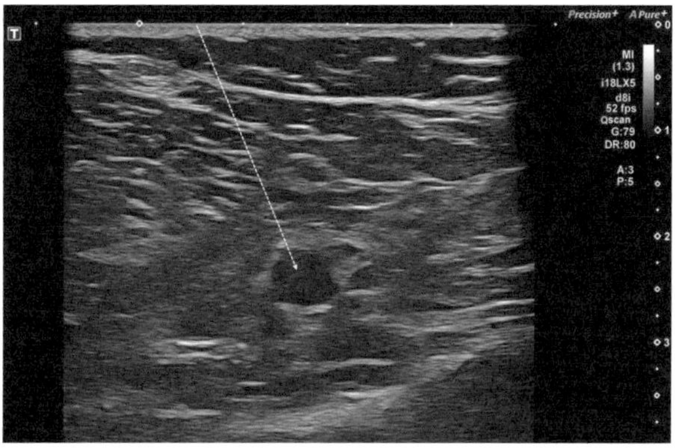

Fig. 3.9 Needle entry path in an oblique out-of-plane access (dotted arrow) avoiding the compressed popliteal vein

Jumper's Knee (Patellar Tendonitis)

Introduction

Jumper's knee, also known as patellar tendonitis, is a condition characterized by inflammation and degeneration of the patellar tendon, which connects the kneecap (patella) to the shinbone (tibia). It is a common overuse injury, particularly among athletes participating in sports that involve repetitive jumping, running, or rapid directional changes, such as basketball, volleyball, or track and field [28].

Epidemiology

Jumper's knee predominantly affects active individuals and athletes, especially those involved in high-impact sports requiring repetitive knee extension. It is reported to occur in 14–20% of athletes participating in jumping sports. The condition is most prevalent among young, active individuals, particularly men aged 16 to 40. Risk factors include repetitive loading of the patellar tendon, participation in sports involving frequent jumping or abrupt stopping and starting, poor biomechanics such as flat feet or tight quadriceps, and inadequate warm-up or muscle conditioning [29–31].

Clinical Presentation and Symptoms

Jumper's knee typically presents with symptoms localized to the patellar tendon. Pain is the hallmark symptom, occurring at the front of the knee, just below the kneecap at the tendon insertion. It is often exacerbated by activities involving knee extension, such as jumping, running, or climbing stairs. In severe cases, the pain may progress to being present even at rest. Tenderness is commonly noted over the patellar tendon, particularly at its attachment to the inferior pole of the patella.

Morning stiffness or stiffness following periods of inactivity is also frequent, along with mild localized swelling along the tendon. Weakness in knee extension may be evident, reducing the ability to perform explosive or weight-bearing movements. These symptoms can lead to functional limitations, impacting athletic performance and daily activities [31–34].

Pathophysiology

Jumper's knee develops as a result of repetitive microtrauma to the patellar tendon, leading to inflammation and, in chronic cases, degenerative changes. Repeated stress causes microtears in the collagen fibers of the tendon, triggering an inflammatory response with the release of cytokines and prostaglandins, resulting in pain and swelling. Chronic tendinosis occurs when continued strain disrupts the healing process, leading to tendon degeneration without significant inflammation. This degeneration is characterized by disorganized collagen fibers, increased proteoglycan deposition, and the formation of abnormal new blood vessels (neovascularization). Hypervascularity contributes to chronic pain and impaired tendon function, while biomechanical overload from abnormal alignment, muscle imbalances, or poor movement patterns exacerbates strain on the tendon [30, 35–38].

Treatment Options

Management of jumper's knee focuses on reducing pain, promoting tendon healing, and preventing recurrence [39–43]:

- *Non-Pharmacological*:
  - *Rest and Activity Modification*:
    Avoid activities that exacerbate symptoms
    Gradual return to activity once pain subsides
  - *Physical Therapy*:
    Eccentric strengthening exercises to promote tendon remodeling
    Stretching of the quadriceps, hamstrings, and calf muscles to relieve tension on the patellar tendon
  - *Cryotherapy*:
    Ice application to reduce pain and inflammation in the acute phase
  - *Bracing or Taping*:
    Patellar straps or kinesiology tape to offload the patellar tendon
  - *Biomechanical Correction*:
    Custom orthotics or footwear adjustments to address underlying gait abnormalities

- *Pharmacological*:
  - NSAIDs for short-term relief of pain and inflammation
  - Topical anti-inflammatory agents for localized symptom management
- *Procedural/Surgical*:
  - Extracorporeal shockwave therapy (ESWT) to stimulate tendon healing
  - Platelet-rich plasma (PRP) injections to promote tendon repair
  - Percutaneous needle tenotomy to release degenerated tissue and encourage healing
  - Surgical debridement for refractory cases to remove degenerated tissue and stimulate regeneration
- *Emerging Therapies*:
  - Stem cell therapy for regenerative healing of the tendon
  - Biologic agents targeting specific inflammatory pathways in chronic cases

In conclusion, jumper's knee is a common overuse injury among athletes, particularly those involved in jumping sports. Early intervention with rest, physical therapy, and biomechanical correction is critical to prevent progression to chronic tendinosis. For severe or refractory cases, advanced therapies such as PRP and shockwave therapy offer promising outcomes.

Dochu algorithm: jumper's knee	
External landmarks	Palpation of the pulsating popliteal artery in the popliteal fossa
Probe positioning	Transverse probe orientation over the popliteal artery with a medial-oblique needle entry (Fig. 3.10)
Target vessel	Popliteal artery (Figs. 3.11 and 3.12)
Needle size	25G, length: 38–62 mm
Medication	Imipenem/Cilastatin (1 vial: 0.5 g/0.5 g) diluted with 10 cc of saline
Dosage	5–10 ml
Cuff position	Lower leg
Cuff compression duration	Deflate cuff 30 s after injection

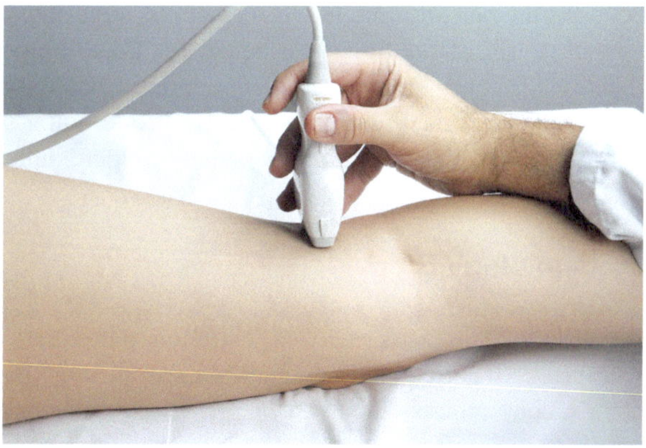

Fig. 3.10 Transverse probe orientation over the palpable popliteal artery approx. 3 cm proximal to the fibular head

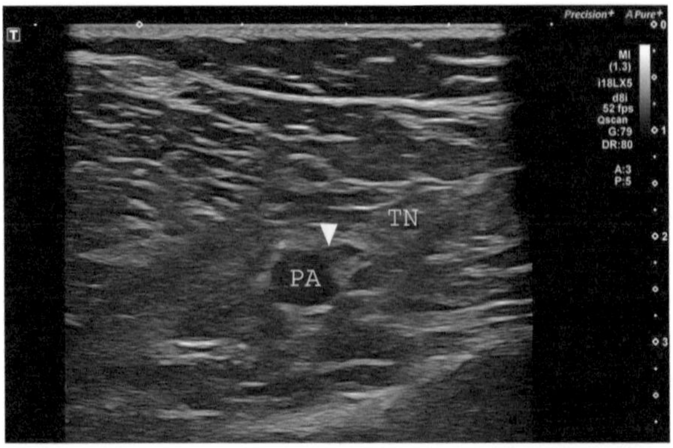

Fig. 3.11 Using compression, the popliteal artery (PA) can be depicted at the level of the popliteal fossa. Compressed popliteal vein (arrowhead). Tibial nerve (TN)

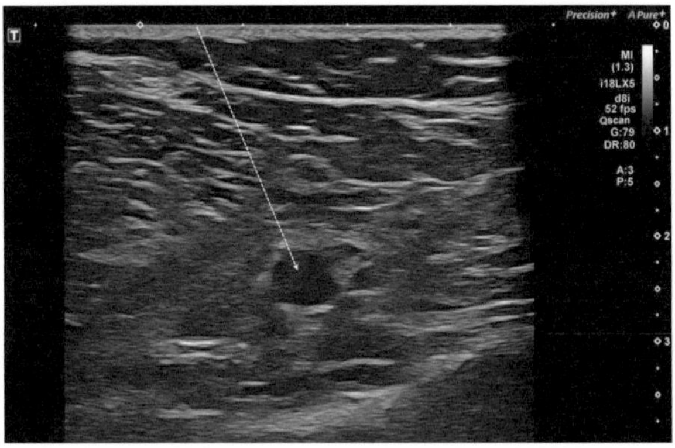

Fig. 3.12 Needle entry path in an oblique out-of-plane access (dotted arrow) avoiding the compressed popliteal vein

Pes Anserine Bursitis

Introduction

Pes anserine bursitis is an inflammatory condition affecting the bursa situated between the pes anserine tendons (gracilis, sartorius, and semitendinosus) and the medial aspect of the tibia, just below the knee joint. This condition results from repetitive friction, trauma, or overuse and is often associated with knee osteoarthritis or biomechanical abnormalities. It is a common source of medial knee pain, particularly in athletes and middle-aged or older adults [44].

Epidemiology

Pes anserine bursitis is relatively common, particularly in individuals with specific risk factors. It is frequently diagnosed in people with knee osteoarthritis and is prevalent among athletes involved in activities requiring running, jumping, or lateral movements [44, 45]. The condition is more common in women, particularly those who are middle-aged, older, or obese. Athletes, especially runners, are also at increased risk. Contributing factors include obesity, which increases load on the knee joint; overuse or repetitive activities such as running or squatting; tightness or weakness in the hamstrings or adductors; and underlying conditions like knee osteoarthritis or diabetes mellitus. Poor biomechanics, such as valgus knee deformity (knock knees), also increase the likelihood of developing this condition [45].

Clinical Presentation and Symptoms

Patients with pes anserine bursitis typically experience localized pain and functional impairment. Pain is the hallmark symptom, localized to the medial knee, approximately 2–4 cm below the joint line on the inner side of the tibia. The pain is often aggravated by activities such as climbing stairs, squatting, or rising from a seated position. In severe cases, pain may occur during rest or at night. Point tenderness is commonly noted over the pes anserine bursa upon palpation, and mild localized swelling in the medial knee region may also be present. Patients may report stiffness or tightness in the medial knee or hamstrings, particularly in the morning or after prolonged inactivity. Functional limitations, including difficulty performing weight-bearing or dynamic activities like running, jumping, or squatting, are also common [44, 46].

Pathophysiology

Pes anserine bursitis is primarily caused by mechanical stress and inflammation. Repetitive friction between the pes anserine tendons and the underlying medial tibia irritates the bursa, leading to inflammation and resulting in pain, swelling, and stiffness. Biomechanical abnormalities, such as valgus knee deformities or poor alignment, exacerbate stress on the medial knee and increase friction. Inflammation triggers hypervascularity, with increased blood vessel proliferation in the bursa, contributing to localized swelling and warmth. Conditions such as knee osteoarthritis or tight hamstrings increase tension on the pes anserine tendons, further predisposing the bursa to inflammation [44].

Treatment Options

Management of pes anserine bursitis focuses on reducing inflammation, alleviating pain, and addressing underlying biomechanical factors [44, 47–50]:

- *Non-Pharmacological*:
  - *Rest and Activity Modification*:
    Avoid activities that exacerbate symptoms, such as running or squatting

- *Ice Therapy*:
  Apply ice packs to reduce inflammation and pain
- *Physical Therapy*:
  Stretching exercises for hamstrings and adductors to reduce tension on the pes anserine tendons
  Strengthening exercises for the quadriceps and core to improve knee stability. Focus on correcting gait abnormalities or biomechanical issues
- *Weight Management*:
  Reducing body weight to decrease stress on the knee joint
- *Supportive Measures*:
  Use of knee braces or padding to provide support and reduce friction

• *Pharmacological*:
  - NSAIDs for pain relief and inflammation control
  - Topical anti-inflammatory agents for localized symptom management
  - Corticosteroid injections into the bursa for severe or persistent inflammation
• *Procedural/Surgical*:
  - Aspiration of the bursa in cases of significant swelling
  - Surgical bursectomy for chronic or recurrent cases unresponsive to conservative management
• *Emerging Therapies*:
  - Platelet-rich plasma (PRP) injections for tendon and bursa healing
  - Ultrasound-guided therapies for precision in treatment delivery

In conclusion, pes anserine bursitis is a common cause of medial knee pain that can significantly impact mobility and quality of life. Early diagnosis and intervention, including physical therapy and biomechanical correction, are critical to managing symptoms and preventing recurrence. For refractory cases, advanced therapeutic options provide promising outcomes.

Dochu algorithm: pes anserine bursitis	
External landmarks	Palpation of the pulsating popliteal artery in the popliteal fossa
Probe positioning	Transverse probe orientation over the popliteal artery with a medial-oblique needle entry (Fig. 3.13)
Target vessel	Popliteal artery (Figs. 3.14 and 3.15)
Needle size	25G, length: 38–62 mm
Medication	Imipenem/Cilastatin (1 vial: 0.5 g/0.5 g) diluted with 10 cc of saline
Dosage	5–10 ml
Cuff position	Lower leg
Cuff compression duration	Deflate cuff 30 s after injection

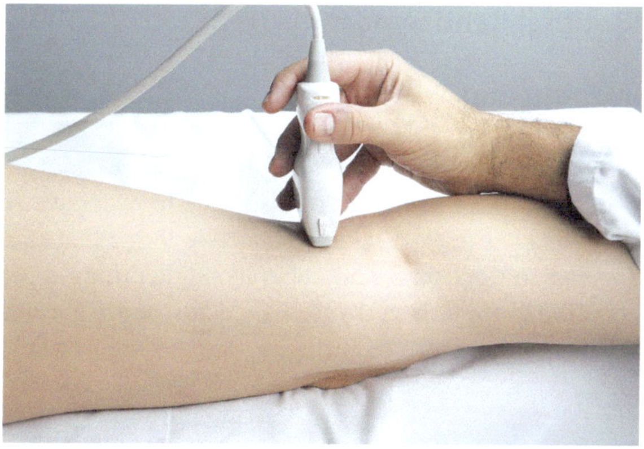

Fig. 3.13 Transverse probe orientation over the palpable popliteal artery approx. 3 cm proximal to the fibular head

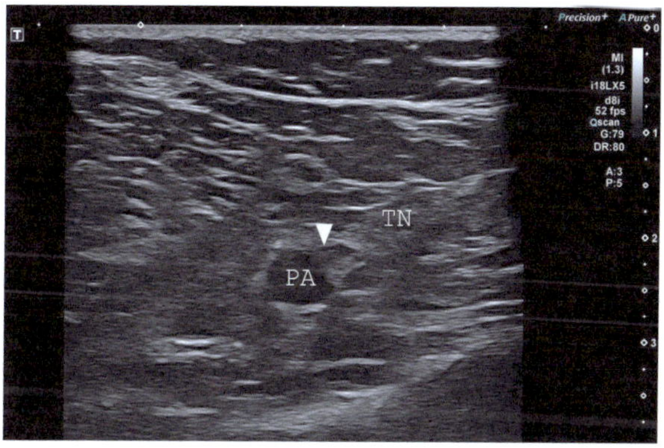

Fig. 3.14 Using compression, the popliteal artery (PA) can be depicted at the level of the popliteal fossa. Compressed popliteal vein (arrowhead). Tibial nerve (TN)

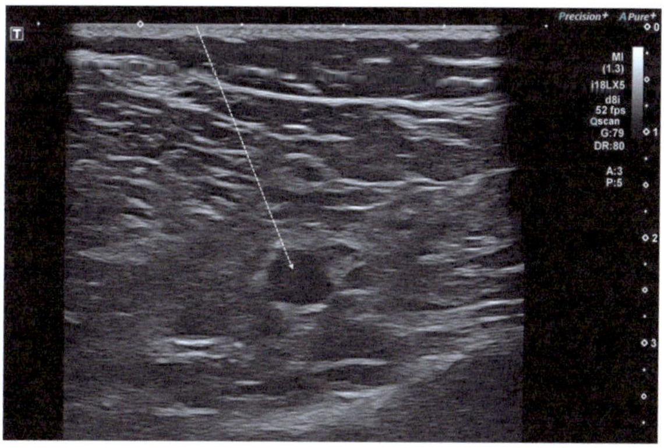

Fig. 3.15 Needle entry path in an oblique out-of-plane access (dotted arrow) avoiding the compressed popliteal vein

Iliotibial Band Syndrome (ITBS)

Introduction

Iliotibial band syndrome (ITBS) is an overuse injury that results in pain along the lateral aspect of the knee. It arises due to excessive friction between the iliotibial (IT) band—a thick band of connective tissue that runs from the hip to the lateral knee—and the lateral femoral epicondyle during repetitive movements. ITBS is a common cause of lateral knee pain, particularly in runners, cyclists, and individuals involved in activities requiring repetitive knee flexion and extension [51, 52].

Epidemiology

ITBS is one of the most prevalent overuse injuries among athletes, particularly runners and cyclists. It accounts for 5–14% of running-related injuries and is also common in cyclists and other athletes who engage in repetitive lower-limb activities. The condition most frequently affects active individuals aged 20 to 40 years. Risk factors include overuse from activities such as running, cycling, or hiking, as well as poor biomechanics, including excessive pronation or leg length discrepancies. Tightness or weakness in the IT band, gluteal muscles, or hip abductors also contributes to the condition, as do sudden increases in training intensity or mileage, inadequate footwear, or inappropriate training surfaces [53–55].

Clinical Presentation and Symptoms

Patients with ITBS typically present with lateral knee pain and related symptoms. The pain is often described as sharp or burning and is localized to the outer side of the knee, near the lateral femoral epicondyle. It tends to worsen with activities such as running downhill, cycling, or prolonged walking, but may subside with rest, only to recur with activity. Point tenderness over the lateral femoral epicondyle is common, and some patients experience mild localized swelling at the site of friction. A snapping sensation over the lateral knee during movement may also be reported. Functional limitations include difficulty continuing physical activities due to pain, and in severe cases, the pain may radiate to the hip or thigh [52, 54, 56].

Pathophysiology

The development of ITBS involves repetitive friction, inflammation, and biomechanical factors. During repetitive knee flexion and extension, the IT band moves over the lateral femoral epicondyle, and excessive motion can irritate and inflame the underlying structures. This friction leads to microtrauma and inflammation of the IT band, periosteum, or adjacent fat pad. Biomechanical contributors, such as weakness or tightness in the gluteal muscles or IT band, alter knee alignment and loading, exacerbating stress on the IT band. Overpronation or improper gait mechanics further increases this strain. Hypervascularity, or increased vascular proliferation in response to inflammation, contributes to pain and swelling [51, 57, 58].

Treatment Options

Treatment of ITBS focuses on reducing inflammation, addressing biomechanical issues, and preventing recurrence [51, 52, 57–61]:

- *Non-Pharmacological*:
  - *Rest and Activity Modification*:
    Avoid activities that aggravate symptoms, such as running or cycling.
    Gradual return to activity after symptoms improve.
  - *Stretching and Foam Rolling*:
    Stretching exercises for the IT band, quadriceps, hamstrings, and hip flexors
    Foam rolling to release tension and reduce tightness in the IT band
  - *Physical Therapy*:
    Strengthening exercises for the gluteal muscles, hip abductors, and core to improve alignment and stability
    Gait retraining to address biomechanical issues
  - *Ice Therapy*:
    Apply ice packs to the lateral knee to reduce inflammation and pain
  - *Footwear and Orthotics*:
    Proper footwear to support the foot and improve alignment
    Custom orthotics for patients with overpronation or leg length discrepancies
- *Pharmacological*:
  - NSAIDs for pain relief and to reduce inflammation
  - Topical anti-inflammatory agents for localized symptom management.
- *Procedural/Surgical*:
  Corticosteroid injections for persistent inflammation and pain
  Surgical release of the IT band or bursectomy in rare, refractory cases
- *Emerging Therapies*:
  - Platelet-rich plasma (PRP) injections to promote healing in chronic cases
  - Shockwave therapy to stimulate tissue repair and reduce pain
  - Stem cell therapy for regenerative healing

In conclusion, ITBS is a common overuse injury that can significantly impact athletic performance and daily activities. Early recognition and treatment with activity modification, physical therapy, and biomechanical corrections are essential for symptom resolution and prevention of recurrence. Advanced therapies provide promising options for patients with chronic or refractory cases.

Dochu algorithm: iliotibial band syndrome	
External landmarks	Palpation of the pulsating popliteal artery in the popliteal fossa
Probe positioning	Transverse probe orientation over the popliteal artery with a medial-oblique needle entry (Fig. 3.16)
Target vessel	Popliteal artery (Figs. 3.17 and 3.18)
Needle size	25G, length: 38–62 mm
Medication	Imipenem/Cilastatin (1 vial: 0.5 g/0.5 g) diluted with 10 cc of saline)
Dosage	5–10 ml
Cuff position	Lower leg
Cuff compression duration	Deflate cuff 30 s after injection

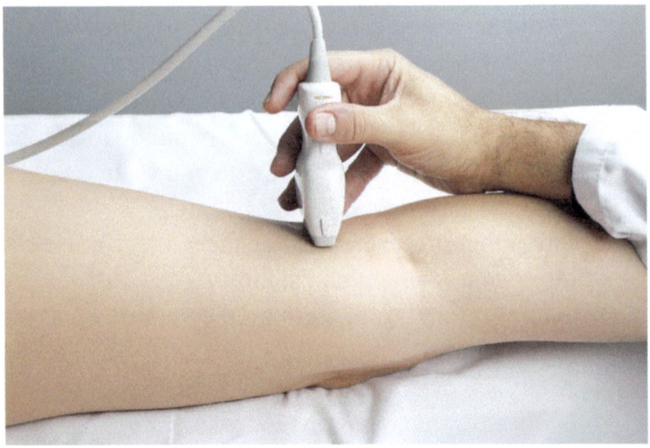

Fig. 3.16 Transverse probe orientation over the palpable popliteal artery approx. 3 cm proximal to the fibular head

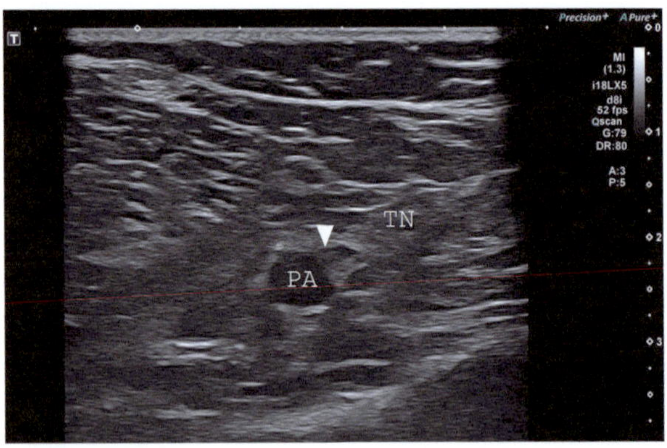

Fig. 3.17 Using compression, the popliteal artery (PA) can be depicted at the level of the popliteal fossa. Compressed popliteal vein (arrowhead). Tibial nerve (TN)

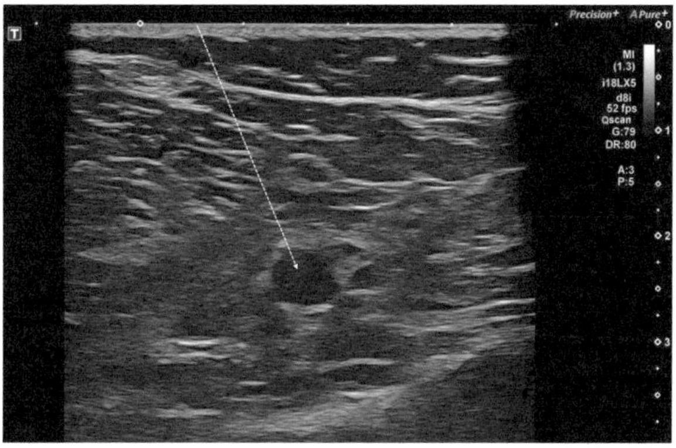

Fig. 3.18 Needle entry path in an oblique out-of-plane access (dotted arrow) avoiding the compressed popliteal vein

Ankle Sprain

Introduction

An ankle sprain is a common musculoskeletal injury that occurs when the ligaments supporting the ankle joint are stretched or torn, typically due to sudden twisting or rolling of the foot. It is one of the most frequent sports-related injuries but can also happen during everyday activities. Most ankle sprains involve the lateral ligaments, particularly the anterior talofibular ligament (ATFL), as a result of the foot rolling inward (inversion) [62].

Epidemiology

Ankle sprains are among the most prevalent orthopedic injuries worldwide, accounting for up to 40% of sports-related injuries. Approximately two million cases are reported annually in the United States alone. They are most common in adolescents and young adults involved in physical activities, particularly athletes participating in sports that require quick changes in direction, such as basketball, football, or tennis. Risk factors include poor proprioception or balance, weak ankle or lower leg muscles, a history of previous ankle sprains (which increases the likelihood of reinjury), wearing inappropriate footwear, and walking on uneven surfaces [63–65].

Clinical Presentation and Symptoms

Ankle sprains are classified into three grades based on severity, each presenting with distinct symptoms. Grade I sprains are mild, involving stretching or minor tearing of the ligaments. Symptoms include mild swelling and tenderness around the ankle, minimal loss of function or instability, and the ability to bear weight with slight discomfort. Grade II sprains are moderate and characterized by partial tearing of the ligaments, moderate swelling, bruising, tenderness, difficulty bearing weight or walking, reduced range of motion, and mild joint instability. Grade III sprains are severe, involving complete ligament tears, significant swelling and bruising, severe pain, inability to bear weight, and marked instability of the ankle joint [66, 67].

Associated symptoms for all grades may include pain at the site of the injured ligament, which worsens with movement or pressure, limited range of motion, and stiffness caused by swelling [66, 67].

Pathophysiology

An ankle sprain results from an acute injury to the ligaments caused by excessive mechanical stress. Sudden inversion or eversion of the foot forces the ligaments to stretch beyond their normal range, leading to microtears or, in severe cases, complete rupture. The injury triggers an inflammatory response, releasing pro-inflammatory cytokines that cause swelling, redness, and pain. Increased vascular permeability leads to fluid accumulation around the injured area, resulting in edema. Ligament healing occurs in three phases: the inflammatory phase, which aims to limit further damage and clear debris; the proliferative phase, where fibroblasts produce new collagen fibers; and the remodeling phase, during which collagen fibers reorganize and strengthen over weeks to months [62, 68, 69].

Treatment Options

Management of an ankle sprain depends on the severity of the injury and focuses on reducing pain, controlling inflammation, and restoring function [68, 70–73]:

- *Acute Phase (First 72 h)*:
  - *RICE Protocol*:
    Rest: Avoid weight-bearing activities to prevent further injury.
    Ice: Apply ice packs for 15–20 min every 1–2 h to reduce swelling and pain.
    Compression: Use an elastic bandage or brace to control swelling and support the joint.
    Elevation: Keep the ankle elevated above heart level to minimize swelling.
- *Non-Pharmacological*:
  - *Physical Therapy*:
    Range-of-motion and stretching exercises to prevent stiffness
    Strengthening exercises for ankle and calf muscles to restore stability
    Balance and proprioception training to reduce the risk of reinjury
  - *Bracing or Taping*:
    Use ankle braces or taping techniques to provide support during activity.
  - *Gradual Return to Activity*:
    Progressive loading and activity modification to avoid overstressing the healing ligaments

- *Pharmacological*:
  - NSAIDs for short-term pain relief and to reduce inflammation
  - Topical analgesics for localized pain management
- *Procedural/Surgical*:
  - *Grade III Sprains*:
    Rarely, surgical repair of torn ligaments may be necessary for severe cases with persistent instability.
    Arthroscopic surgery to address associated injuries, such as cartilage damage
  - *Immobilization*:
    Use of a walking boot or cast for severe sprains
- *Emerging Therapies*:
  - Platelet-rich plasma (PRP) injections to promote ligament healing
  - Ultrasound-guided therapies for precision treatment of ligament injuries
  - Stem cell therapy for enhanced tissue repair in chronic or recurrent cases

Rehabilitation and Prevention

Rehabilitation focuses on restoring ankle function and preventing future sprains:

- *Rehabilitation*:
  - Gradual reintroduction of weight-bearing and functional activities
  - Plyometric exercises to improve dynamic stability for athletes
- *Prevention*:
  - Regular strength and balance training
  - Wearing appropriate footwear during activities
  - Use of ankle braces or taping for individuals with a history of recurrent sprains

In conclusion, ankle sprains are common injuries that range in severity from mild ligament stretching to complete tears. Prompt treatment using the RICE protocol, followed by structured rehabilitation, can ensure a full recovery. Advanced therapies and surgical interventions may be necessary for severe or recurrent cases, with a focus on restoring stability and preventing chronic instability.

Dochu algorithm: ankle sprains	
External landmarks	Palpaple tendon of the extensor hallucis longus muscle, palpable dorsal pedal artery
Probe positioning	Transverse probe orientation over the extensor halluces longus tendon at the level of the intermalleolar line (Fig. 3.19)
Target vessel	Dorsal pedal artery (Figs. 3.20 and 3.21)
Needle size	27G, length: 19 mm
Medication	Imipenem/Cilastatin (1 vial: 0.5 g/0.5 g) diluted with 10 cc of saline
Dosage	1.5 ml
Cuff position	Distal foot
Cuff compression duration	Deflate cuff 30 s after injection

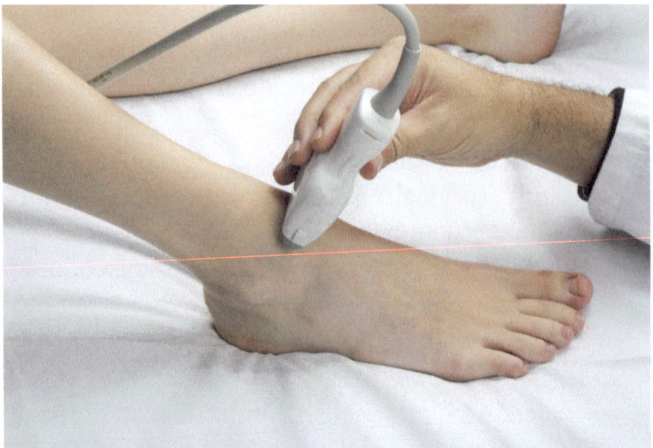

Fig. 3.19 Transverse probe orientation at the level of the intermalleolar line over the palpable dorsal pedal artery

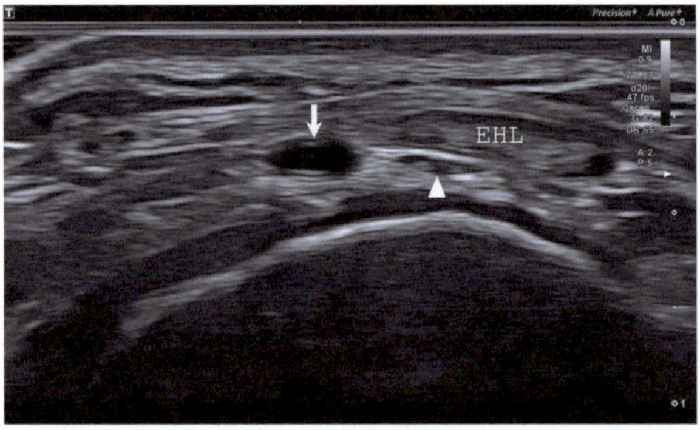

Fig. 3.20 Depiction of the dorsal pedal artery (arrow) lateral to the extensor hallucis longus tendon (EHL). Deep fibular nerve (arrowhead)

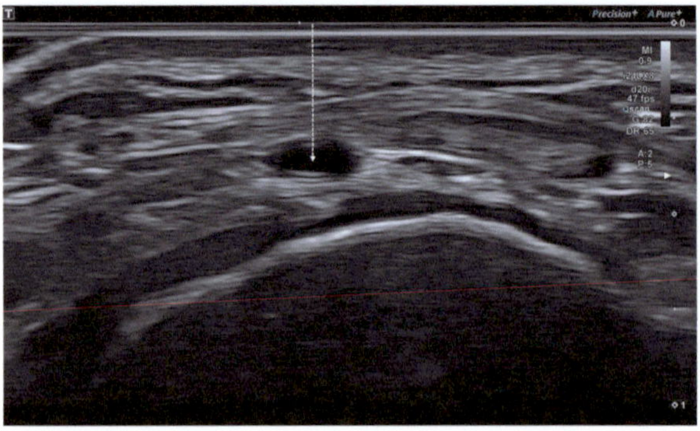

Fig. 3.21 Needle entry path in an out-of-plane access (dotted arrow)

Ankle Osteoarthritis (OA)

Introduction

Ankle osteoarthritis (OA) is a degenerative joint condition characterized by the progressive deterioration of cartilage in the tibiotalar joint, resulting in pain, stiffness, and functional limitations. Unlike osteoarthritis of the knee or hip, which is often idiopathic, ankle OA is frequently post-traumatic, developing as a result of previous fractures, ligament injuries, or repeated stress on the joint. This condition is a significant cause of disability, particularly in active and aging populations [74, 75].

Epidemiology

Although less common than OA in other weight-bearing joints, ankle OA has a substantial impact on those affected. It is estimated to affect approximately 1–4% of the population, with 70–80% of cases being post-traumatic in origin. The condition is more prevalent in individuals with a history of ankle injuries, and it most commonly occurs in middle-aged and older adults. Key risk factors include trauma, such as previous fractures or repeated ankle sprains, obesity, which increases joint stress and accelerates cartilage wear, and biomechanical abnormalities like varus or valgus deformities. Repetitive strain from occupational or athletic activities involving high-impact motions also contributes to its development [74–76].

Clinical Presentation and Symptoms

Ankle OA typically presents with symptoms associated with joint degeneration. Pain is a primary feature, described as a deep, aching sensation localized to the ankle joint. This pain worsens with weight-bearing activities, such as walking, climbing stairs, or running, and may persist at rest or during the night in advanced cases. Stiffness is common, particularly in the morning or after prolonged inactivity, and often lasts less than 30 min [74, 77].

Patients frequently experience recurrent or persistent swelling around the ankle joint, caused by synovial inflammation or joint effusion. Reduced range of motion is another hallmark symptom, with difficulty dorsiflexing or plantarflexing the ankle, as well as challenges navigating uneven terrain or stairs. Crepitus, a grinding or cracking sensation during movement, may occur due to cartilage loss, and in severe cases, visible deformities such as varus or valgus alignment changes can develop. Functional limitations, including difficulty walking long distances or performing activities requiring ankle mobility, are also common [78, 79].

Pathophysiology

The progression of ankle OA involves a combination of mechanical stress, cartilage degeneration, and inflammatory processes. Repeated mechanical loading leads to microdamage in the articular cartilage, resulting in progressive thinning and exposure of the subchondral bone. This increased friction contributes to joint pain and promotes subchondral bone changes, such as sclerosis and cyst formation [80, 81].

Osteophytes, or bone spurs, often develop at the margins of the joint, further limiting motion and exacerbating pain. Cartilage debris triggers synovial inflammation, characterized by the release of cytokines like interleukin-1 (IL-1) and tumor necrosis factor-alpha (TNF-α), which sustain the inflammatory response. Hypervascularity, or increased blood vessel proliferation in the synovium, contributes to persistent swelling, warmth, and inflammation. As cartilage loss progresses, joint space narrows, resulting in mechanical instability [82, 83].

Treatment Options

Treatment for ankle OA focuses on pain management, restoring function, and preventing further joint degeneration [74, 84–87]:

- *Non-Pharmacological*:
  - *Lifestyle Modifications*:
    Weight management to reduce stress on the ankle joint
    Activity modification to avoid high-impact activities
  - *Physical Therapy*:
    Range-of-motion exercises to maintain flexibility
    Strengthening exercises for the lower leg and ankle muscles to support the joint
    Balance and proprioception training to improve stability
  - *Footwear and Orthotics*:
    Use of cushioned shoes or custom orthotics to improve joint alignment and shock absorption
    Ankle braces or supports for stability
- *Pharmacological*:
  - NSAIDs for pain relief and inflammation control
  - Topical analgesics like capsaicin or diclofenac gel for localized symptom management
  - Corticosteroid injections for acute flare-ups of inflammation
  - Hyaluronic acid injections to improve joint lubrication and reduce pain (limited evidence in the ankle compared to the knee)
- *Procedural/Surgical*:
  - *Arthroscopic Debridement*:
    Removal of loose cartilage or bone fragments in mild to moderate cases
  - *Osteotomy*:

Realignment surgery to redistribute joint load in cases of malalignment
  - *Ankle Arthrodesis (Fusion)*:
    Fusion of the tibia and talus bones to eliminate pain in advanced cases, though at the cost of mobility
  - *Total Ankle Replacement*:
    Prosthetic replacement of the joint to restore motion and relieve pain in select patients
- *Emerging Therapies*:
  - Platelet-rich plasma (PRP) injections for cartilage repair and anti-inflammatory effects
  - Stem cell therapy to promote regeneration of damaged cartilage
  - Biologic agents targeting inflammatory cytokines

In conclusion, ankle OA is a challenging condition that significantly impacts mobility and quality of life. Early intervention with lifestyle changes, physical therapy, and pharmacological measures can slow disease progression. For severe cases, surgical and emerging regenerative therapies offer promising solutions for improved long-term outcomes.

Dochu algorithm: ankle osteoarthritis	
External landmarks	Palpaple tendon of the extensor hallucis longus muscle, palpable dorsal pedal artery
Probe positioning	Transverse probe orientation over the extensor hallucis longus tendon at the level of the intermalleolar line (Fig. 3.22)
Target vessel	Dorsal pedal artery (Figs. 3.23 and 3.24)
Needle size	27G, length: 19 mm
Medication	Imipenem/Cilastatin (1 vial: 0.5 g/0.5 g) diluted with 10 cc of saline
Dosage	1.5 ml
Cuff position	Distal foot
Cuff compression duration	Deflate cuff 30 s after injection

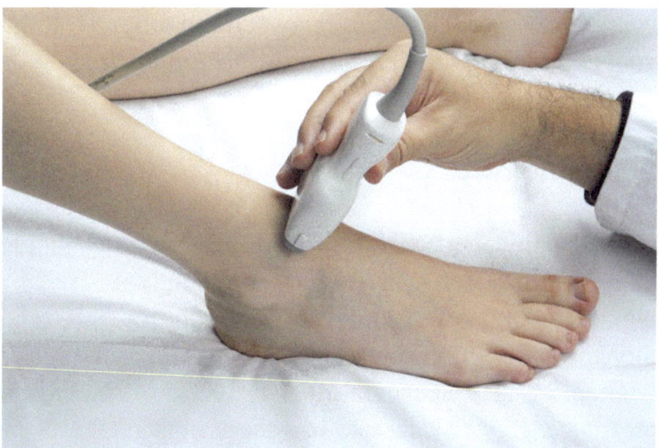

Fig. 3.22 Transverse probe orientation at the level of the intermalleolar line over the palpable dorsal pedal artery

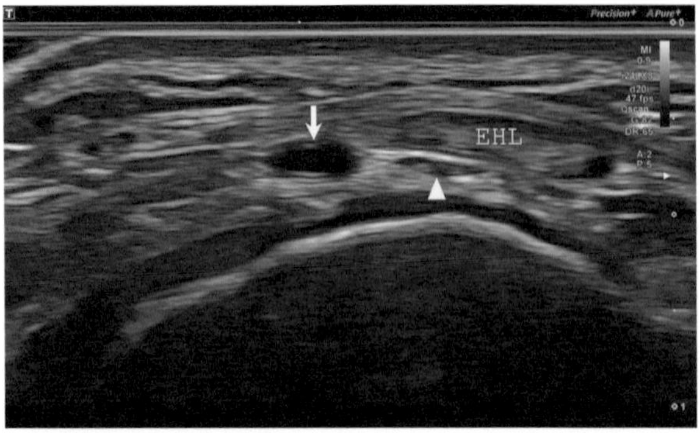

Fig. 3.23 Depiction of the dorsal pedal artery (arrow) lateral to the extensor hallucis longus tendon (EHL). Deep fibular nerve (arrowhead)

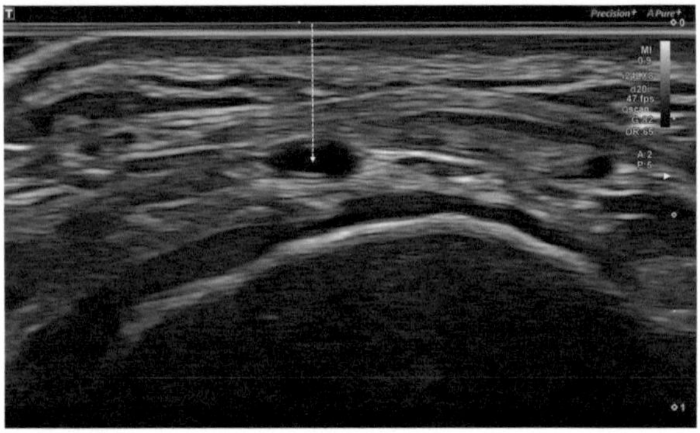

Fig. 3.24 Needle entry path in an out-of-plane access (dotted arrow)

Gout—Foot and Ankle

Introduction

Gout is a form of inflammatory arthritis caused by the deposition of monosodium urate (MSU) crystals in joints due to hyperuricemia, which is elevated serum uric acid levels. This condition is characterized by sudden and severe episodes of joint pain, redness, and swelling, most commonly affecting the big toe. If left untreated, gout can progress to chronic arthritis, joint deformity, and kidney damage [88, 89].

Epidemiology

Gout is a prevalent condition worldwide, with its incidence rising due to changes in diet and lifestyle. It affects approximately 1–4% of the global population, with higher rates observed in developed countries [90, 91]. The condition is more common in men, with peak onset occurring between the ages of 30 and 50. Postmenopausal women are also at increased risk due to hormonal changes that impair uric acid clearance. Key risk factors include a high intake of purine-rich foods such as red meat and seafood, as well as alcohol consumption, particularly beer. Metabolic conditions such as obesity, metabolic syndrome, hypertension, and insulin resistance further contribute to the risk. Certain medications, including diuretics, low-dose aspirin, and immunosuppressants like cyclosporine, can also predispose individuals to gout. A family history of gout or hyperuricemia increases susceptibility [89–92].

Clinical Presentation and Symptoms

Gout progresses through four distinct stages, with acute attacks being the most recognizable.

The first stage, asymptomatic hyperuricemia, involves elevated serum uric acid levels without clinical symptoms. This is followed by acute gout flares, characterized by a sudden onset of severe pain, often occurring at night. Common symptoms during this stage include erythema, warmth, and swelling in the affected joint, most frequently the first metatarsophalangeal (MTP) joint of the big toe. Pain peaks within 24 h and may persist for days to weeks. In severe cases, fever and systemic symptoms may also occur [89, 93].

The third stage, intercritical gout, refers to asymptomatic periods between acute flares. However, during these intervals, urate crystals continue to deposit in joints and tissues, potentially leading to future complications. In the final stage, chronic tophaceous gout, patients experience persistent joint pain and stiffness. Tophi, which are visible deposits of urate crystals, may form in joints, tendons, and soft tissues. This stage can result in joint deformity and reduced function in advanced cases [89, 93].

Pathophysiology

Gout arises from the accumulation of monosodium urate crystals in joints, which triggers a potent inflammatory response. Hyperuricemia occurs due to overproduction, decreased excretion of uric acid, or a combination of both. When uric acid levels exceed their solubility limit, MSU crystals precipitate in the synovial fluid, particularly in cooler peripheral joints. These crystals activate the innate immune system by engaging the NLRP3 inflammasome, leading to the release of pro-inflammatory cytokines such as interleukin-1β (IL-1β). This, in turn, recruits neutrophils and initiates acute inflammation [94].

Repeated flares and ongoing crystal deposition cause chronic damage, including cartilage degradation, joint erosion, and the formation of tophi. Increased vascularity in the synovium during acute attacks further contributes to the redness, warmth, and swelling associated with gout [88, 89].

Treatment Options

Management of gout aims to relieve acute flares, prevent future attacks, and lower serum uric acid levels [95–99]:

- *Acute Gout Flares*:
  - *NSAIDs*: Indomethacin, naproxen, or ibuprofen for pain and inflammation
  - *Colchicine*: Effective for reducing inflammation when taken early
  - *Corticosteroids*: Prednisone or intra-articular injections for severe attacks or NSAID contraindications
- *Long-Term Management*:
  - *Urate-Lowering Therapy (ULT)*:
    Allopurinol (xanthine oxidase inhibitor) to reduce uric acid production
    Febuxostat for patients intolerant to allopurinol
    Probenecid (uricosuric agent) to enhance uric acid excretion
  - *Lifestyle Modifications*:
    Low-purine diet (avoid red meat, shellfish, alcohol, and sugary drinks)
    Weight management and regular exercise
    Adequate hydration to improve uric acid excretion
- *Chronic Tophaceous Gout*:
  - Surgical removal of large or disabling tophi
  - Advanced imaging (e.g., ultrasound or dual-energy CT) to monitor urate crystal burden
- *Emerging Therapies*:
  - IL-1 inhibitors (e.g., anakinra, canakinumab) for patients with frequent flares or contraindications to standard therapies
  - Pegloticase (recombinant uricase) for refractory cases

In conclusion, gout is a complex and increasingly common condition that requires a multifaceted approach for effective management. Early intervention during acute attacks and sustained urate-lowering strategies are critical to prevent complications and improve long-term outcomes. Advances in biologics and novel therapies offer promising options for refractory and chronic cases.

Dochu algorithm: gout (foot and ankle)	
External landmarks	1. Palpaple tendon of the extensor hallucis longus muscle, palpable dorsal pedal artery 2. Palpaple malleolus medialis
Probe positioning	1. Transverse probe orientation over the extensor hallucis longus tendon at the level of the intermalleolar line (Fig. 3.25) 2. Transverse probe orientation dorsal and approx. 1 cm cranial to the medial malleolus. (Fig. 3.26). Cave: tibial nerve!
Target vessel	1. Dorsal pedal artery (Figs. 3.27 and 3.28) 2. Posterior tibial artery (Figs. 3.29 and 3.30)
Needle size	27G, length: 19 mm

(continued)

Medication	Imipenem/Cilastatin (1 vial: 0.5 g/0.5 g) diluted with 10 cc of saline
Dosage	1.5 ml each
Cuff position	NA

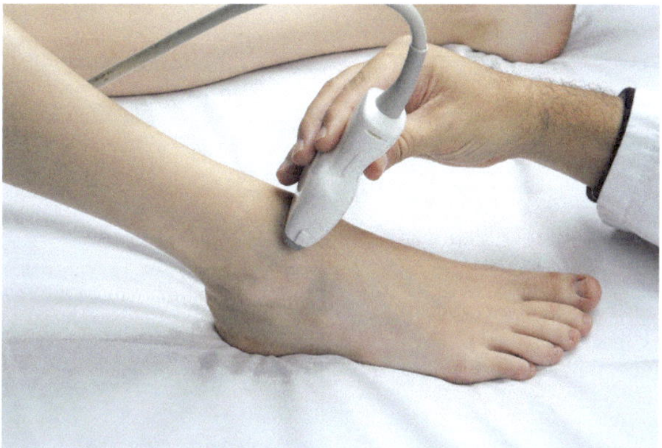

Fig. 3.25 Transverse probe orientation at the level of the intermalleolar line over the palpable dorsal pedal artery

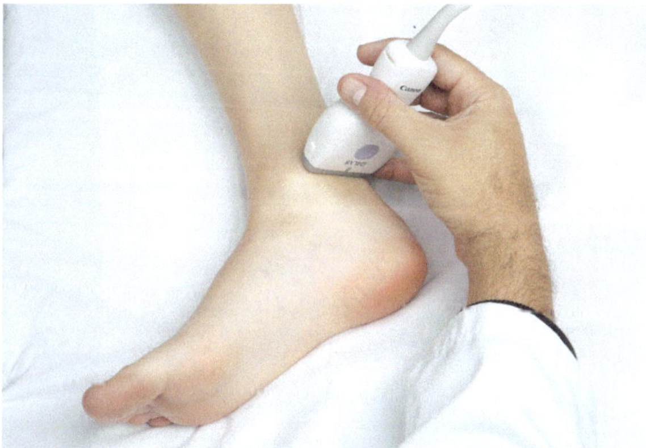

Fig. 3.26 Transverse probe orientation dorsal and approx. 1 cm cranial to the medial malleolus

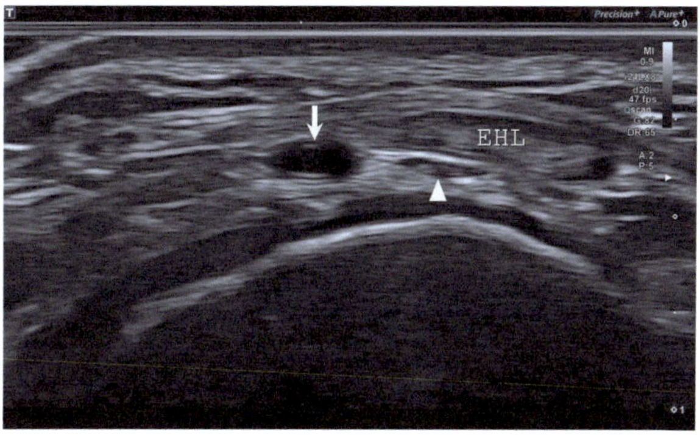

Fig. 3.27 Depiction of the dorsal pedal artery (arrow) lateral to the extensor hallucis longus tendon (EHL). Deep fibular nerve (arrowhead)

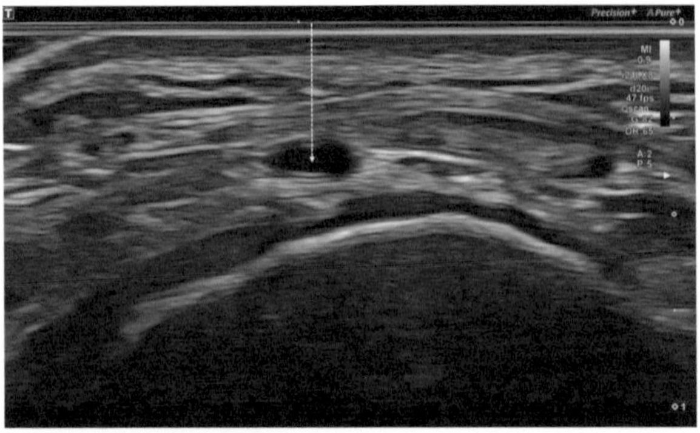

Fig. 3.28 Needle entry path in an out-of-plane access (dotted arrow)

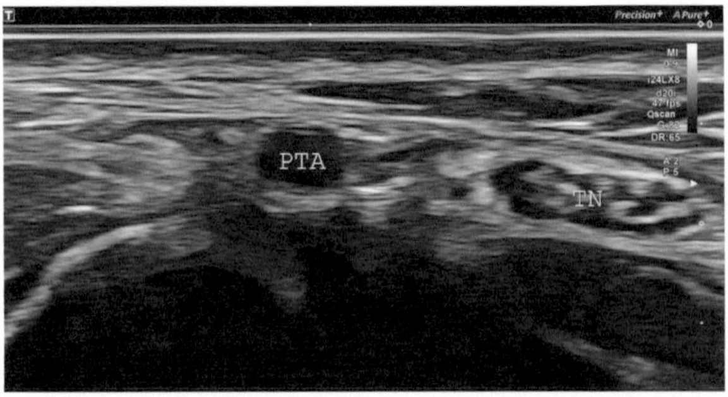

Fig. 3.29 Depiction of the posterior tibial artery (PTA) at the level of the medial malleolus. Tibial nerve (TN)

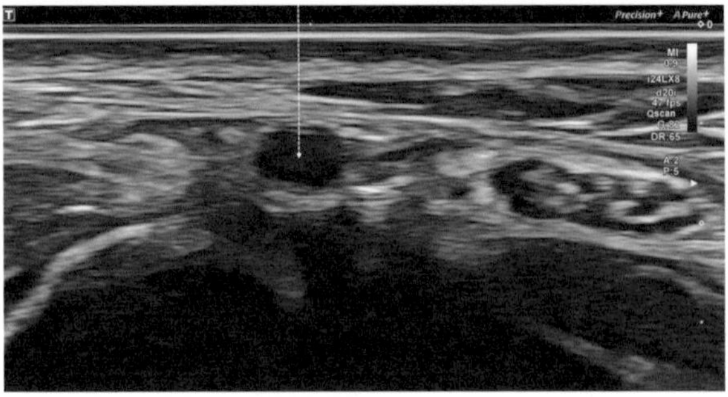

Fig. 3.30 Needle entry path in an out-of-plane access (dotted arrow)

Achilles Tendonitis

Introduction

Achilles tendonitis refers to inflammation of the Achilles tendon, the largest tendon in the body, connecting the calf muscles to the heel bone (calcaneus). This condition is often caused by overuse and repetitive strain, especially in athletes or individuals involved in activities that require running, jumping, or sudden changes in direction. In some cases, chronic Achilles tendonitis can progress to Achilles tendinosis, where the tendon undergoes degenerative changes rather than remaining inflamed [100].

Epidemiology

Achilles tendonitis is a common musculoskeletal disorder, particularly prevalent among active individuals. It accounts for about 6–18% of all injuries related to running. The condition is most commonly observed in people aged 30–50, although it can also affect younger athletes. Various risk factors contribute to the development of Achilles tendonitis, such as participation in sports or activities that involve repetitive ankle motion, including running and basketball. Sudden increases in training intensity or duration, as well as biomechanical issues like flat feet, high arches, or tight calf muscles, also increase the risk. Additionally, inappropriate footwear and systemic factors such as obesity or underlying inflammatory conditions, like rheumatoid arthritis, can further predispose individuals to developing this condition [101].

Clinical Presentation and Symptoms

Individuals with Achilles tendonitis typically present with symptoms that vary depending on the stage and severity of the condition. Pain is often localized along the tendon, either a few centimeters above the heel (mid-portion tendonitis) or at the heel bone itself (insertional tendonitis). The pain tends to worsen with physical activity, particularly during running or climbing stairs, and is often accompanied by stiffness and discomfort, which is most noticeable in the morning or after prolonged periods of inactivity. Swelling or thickening along the affected portion of the tendon may also be present, and in some cases, palpable nodules may form. Tenderness is often felt upon palpation of the tendon, especially when the foot is moved into dorsiflexion or plantarflexion. In certain instances, a grinding or creaking sensation (crepitus) can be felt when the tendon moves. This condition can lead to functional limitations, including difficulty with activities that require pushing off the foot, such as sprinting or jumping.

Pathophysiology

Achilles tendonitis arises from repetitive microtrauma to the tendon, which triggers an inflammatory response. In the acute stage, repetitive strain leads to small tears in the collagen fibers of the tendon, resulting in inflammation. This process involves the release of prostaglandins and cytokines, which mediate the inflammatory response. If the condition becomes chronic, however, it transitions into Achilles tendinosis, where persistent strain and insufficient healing lead to tendon degeneration. The tendon's collagen fibers become disorganized, and increased proteoglycan deposition and vascular proliferation (neovascularization) are observed. Hypervascularity contributes to the pain and delayed healing. Biomechanical factors, such as tight calf muscles or poor ankle flexibility, may exacerbate the tension on the Achilles tendon. Additionally, altered gait mechanics or overpronation can further strain the tendon.

Treatment Options

Effective management of Achilles tendonitis varies depending on the severity and chronicity of the condition:

- *Non-Pharmacological*:
  - Rest and activity modification to reduce repetitive strain on the tendon
  - Ice application to manage pain and inflammation during the acute phase
  - Physical therapy focusing on:
    Eccentric strengthening exercises to promote tendon remodeling
    Stretching of the Achilles tendon and calf muscles to improve flexibility
  - Proper footwear or orthotics to correct biomechanical issues and provide adequate support
- *Pharmacological*:
  - NSAIDs for short-term relief of pain and inflammation in the acute phase
  - Topical anti-inflammatory agents for localized symptom management
- *Procedural/Surgical*:
  - Extracorporeal shock wave therapy (ESWT) to stimulate tendon healing in chronic cases.
  - Percutaneous needle tenotomy to stimulate tissue repair in degenerated tendons
  - Surgical debridement for chronic cases with significant tendon degeneration or persistent symptoms
- *Emerging Therapies*:
  - Platelet-rich plasma (PRP) injections to enhance tendon healing
  - Stem cell therapy to promote regeneration of damaged tendon tissue
  - Biologics targeting inflammatory pathways in cases of systemic inflammatory contributions

In conclusion, Achilles tendonitis is a common overuse injury that can significantly impair mobility and quality of life. Early diagnosis and a multidisciplinary approach involving activity modification, physical therapy, and targeted interventions can lead to successful outcomes. For chronic or refractory cases, advanced regenerative therapies and surgical options offer promising solutions.

Dochu algorithm: achilles tendonitis	
External landmarks	Poplital approach: Palpation of the pulsating popliteal artery in the popliteal fossa
Probe positioning	1. Transverse probe orientation over the popliteal artery with a medial-oblique needle entry (Fig. 3.31)
Target vessel	Popliteal artery (Figs. 3.32 and 3.33)
Needle size	25G, length: 38–62 mm
Medication	Imipenem/Cilastatin (1 vial: 0.5 g/0.5 g) diluted with 10 cc of saline
Dosage	10 ml
Cuff position	Distal foot
Cuff compression duration	Deflate cuff 60 s after injection

*Due to the variable supply of the Achilles tendon (fibular artery, posterior tibial artery, or both) Dochu is recommended on the popliteal artery

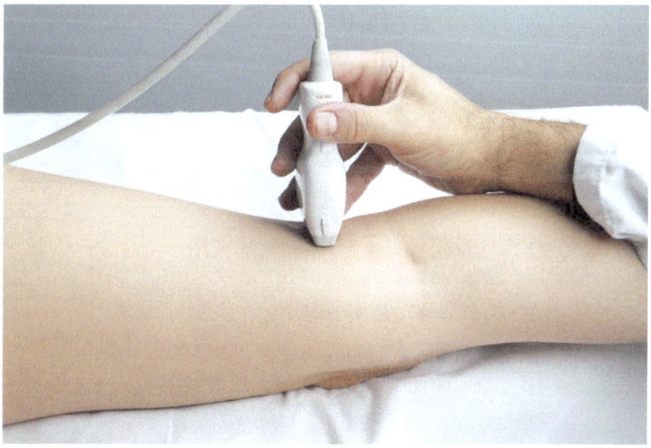

Fig. 3.31 Transverse probe orientation over the palpable popliteal artery approx. 3 cm proximal to the fibular head

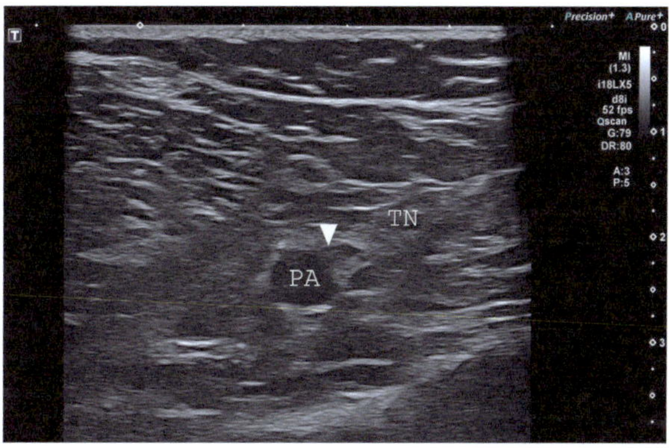

Fig. 3.32 Using compression, the popliteal artery (PA) can be depicted at the level of the popliteal fossa. Compressed popliteal vein (arrowhead). Tibial nerve (TN)

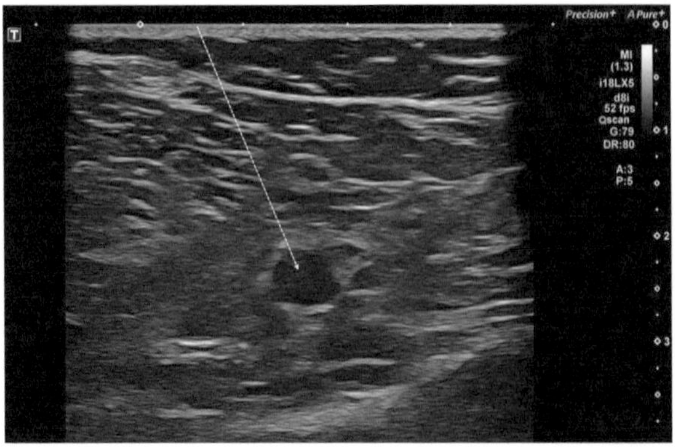

Fig. 3.33 Needle entry path in an oblique out-of-plane access (dotted arrow) avoiding the compressed popliteal vein

Plantar Fasciitis

Introduction

Plantar fasciitis is one of the most common causes of heel pain, resulting from inflammation of the plantar fascia, a thick band of connective tissue that supports the arch of the foot. This condition is often linked to repetitive strain or overuse, leading to microtears in the fascia. It predominantly affects individuals with prolonged weight-bearing activities or those with structural foot abnormalities [102].

Epidemiology

Plantar fasciitis is highly prevalent, especially among active adults and middle-aged individuals. Studies show that approximately 10% of the population will experience plantar fasciitis at some point in their lives, with prevalence being highest amongst those aged between 40 and 60 years old, although it can generally affect people of all ages. Its occurrence is additionally influenced by lifestyle factors.

- *Prevalence*: Affects approximately 10% of the population at some point in their lives
- *Age*: Most common in individuals aged 40–60 years
- *Risk Factors*:
  - Obesity, which increases stress on the plantar fascia
  - Repetitive and demanding activities like running, dancing, or standing for long hours
  - Foot structure abnormalities, such as having flat feet or high arches
  - Use of improper footwear lacking arch cushioning or support

Clinical Presentation and Symptoms

Patients with plantar fasciitis typically present with characteristic symptoms affecting their heel and foot [102, 103, 104]:

- *Pain*:
  - Sharp, stabbing pain at the bottom of the heel, especially upon waking and taking the first few steps of the day (also known as start-up pain)
  - Pain often improves with gradual movement but may worsen after prolonged standing or physical activity.
- *Tenderness*:
  - Palpation reveals tenderness along the medial side of the heel.
- *Stiffness*:
  - Tightness in the plantar fascia or Achilles tendon, particularly after periods of inactivity
- *Swelling*:
  - Mild swelling may be observed in the heel region
- *Functional Limitations*:
  - Difficulty walking, running, or participating in sports

Pathophysiology

The underlying pathophysiology of plantar fasciitis involves repetitive microtrauma and subsequent inflammatory changes in the plantar fascia [104–106]:

- *Mechanical Overload*:
  - Excessive strain leads to microtears in the fascia near its insertion on the calcaneus (heel bone).
- *Inflammatory Response*:
  - Inflammatory mediators, such as prostaglandins and cytokines, are released, causing localized pain and swelling.
- *Hypervascularity*:
  - Increased vascular proliferation occurs as part of the healing response, but chronic overuse disrupts this process, leading to persistent inflammation.
- *Degenerative Changes*:
  - Long-standing plantar fasciitis may progress to degenerative fasciitis, characterized by thickening and fibrosis of the plantar fascia.
- *Association with Tight Muscles*:
  - Tightness in the calf muscles or Achilles tendon exacerbates tension on the plantar fascia, maintaining symptoms.

Treatment Options

Management of plantar fasciitis focuses on alleviating pain, promoting healing, and preventing recurrence [104, 107–109]:

- *Non-Pharmacological*:
  - Rest and avoidance of activities that aggravate the condition
  - Stretching exercises for the plantar fascia and calf muscles
  - Orthotic devices or insoles for arch support and heel cushioning
  - Night splints to maintain the foot in a dorsiflexed position and reduce morning pain
  - Physical therapy to strengthen foot and lower leg muscles
- *Pharmacological*:
  - NSAIDs to manage pain and inflammation
  - Topical analgesics for localized relief
  - Corticosteroid injections for severe or refractory cases
- *Procedural/Surgical*:
  - Extracorporeal shock wave therapy (ESWT) to stimulate healing in chronic cases
  - Plantar fascia release surgery for refractory cases unresponsive to conservative measures.
- *Emerging Therapies*:
  - Platelet-rich plasma (PRP) injections to promote tissue repair.
  - Botox injections to relieve tension in the plantar fascia.

In conclusion, plantar fasciitis is a common yet debilitating condition that significantly impacts mobility and quality of life. A combination of early intervention, lifestyle modifications, and tailored treatment options can help patients achieve pain relief and prevent recurrence. Advances in regenerative therapies offer promising future treatment options for persistent cases.

Dochu algorithm: plantar fasciitis	
External landmarks	Palpaple malleolus medialis
Probe positioning	Transverse probe orientation dorsal and approx. 1 cm cranial to the medial malleolus (Fig. 3.34). Cave: tibial nerve!
Target vessel	Posterior tibial artery (Figs. 3.35 and 3.36)
Needle size	27G, length: 19–25 mm
Medication	Imipenem/Cilastatin (1vial: 0.5 g/0.5 g) diluted with 10 cc of saline
Dosage	1.5 ml
Cuff position	NA

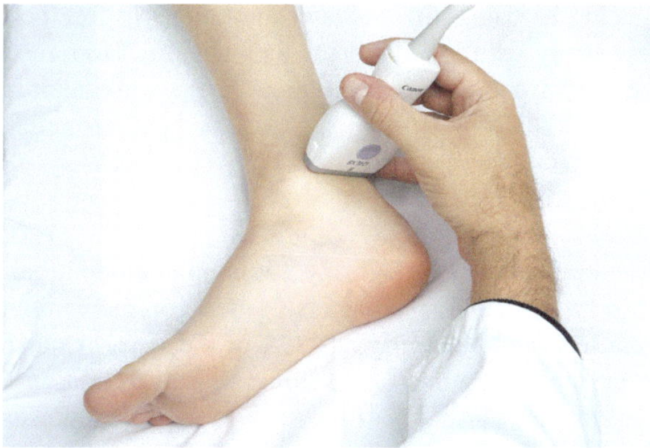

Fig. 3.34 Transverse probe orientation dorsal and approx. 1 cm cranial to the medial malleolus

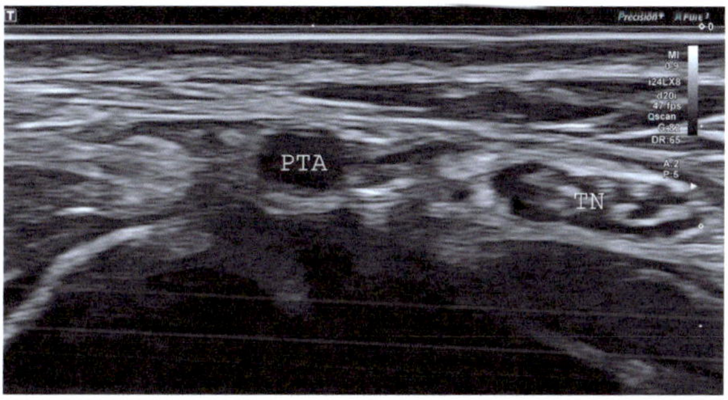

Fig. 3.35 Depiction of the posterior tibial artery (PTA) at the level of the medial malleolus. Tibial nerve (TN)

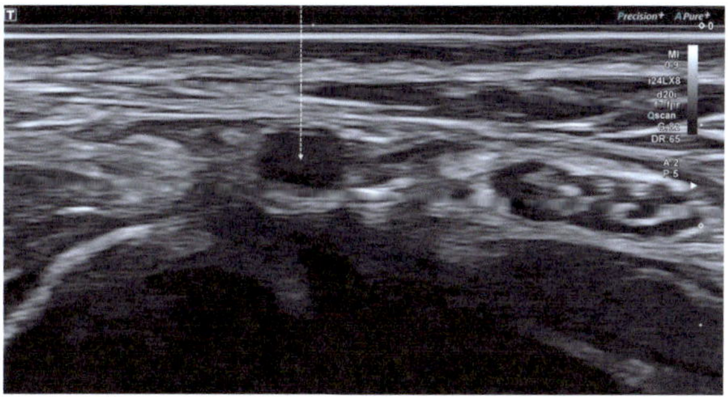

Fig. 3.36 Needle entry path in an out-of-plane access (dotted arrow)

Metatarsal Osteoarthritis (OA)

Introduction

Metatarsal osteoarthritis (OA) is a degenerative condition affecting the joints of the metatarsals, with the first metatarsophalangeal (MTP) joint being the most commonly involved. It is characterized by the progressive breakdown of cartilage, leading to pain, stiffness, and limitations in forefoot function. Metatarsal OA is frequently seen in individuals with abnormal foot mechanics, a history of injuries, or repetitive stress from activities such as walking or sports [110, 111].

Epidemiology

Metatarsal OA is a relatively common condition, particularly in older adults and those with specific risk factors. It most commonly affects the first MTP joint, often referred to as hallux rigidus. OA of the lesser metatarsals is less frequent but can occur due to trauma or systemic arthritic conditions. Women are more likely to develop metatarsal OA, partly due to footwear choices such as high heels, and the condition frequently affects individuals over the age of 50. Risk factors include repetitive stress from activities like running, dancing, or prolonged standing; foot deformities such as bunions, flat feet, or high arches; obesity, which increases load on the metatarsal joints; a history of trauma or fractures; and systemic conditions such as rheumatoid arthritis or gout [112, 113].

Clinical Presentation and Symptoms

Patients with metatarsal OA often present with forefoot symptoms that impair mobility and daily activities. Pain is a common complaint, localized to the metatarsal joints and aggravated by weight-bearing activities. It is typically worse during movement or at the end of the day. Morning stiffness or stiffness after periods of inactivity is also reported, alongside a reduced range of motion, particularly in dorsiflexion of the first MTP joint [77].

Other symptoms include mild to moderate swelling around the affected joints, tenderness upon palpation, and a grinding or popping sensation (crepitus) during joint movement due to cartilage loss. Visible deformities, such as joint enlargement or bony prominences, may be present. In advanced cases, joint misalignment or structural changes can occur. Functional limitations are common, with patients experiencing difficulty walking, running, or wearing certain types of footwear. Pain or discomfort during toe-off in the gait cycle further affects mobility [114, 115].

Pathophysiology

The progression of metatarsal OA involves cartilage degeneration, mechanical overload, and inflammatory processes. Repetitive stress leads to microdamage in the articular cartilage, resulting in the loss of cushioning and increased friction. Progressive cartilage loss causes joint space narrowing, exacerbating stiffness and pain. Bone spurs, or osteophytes, often develop at the joint margins as a compensatory response, limiting joint motion and causing deformity [80, 116].

Subchondral bone changes, including sclerosis and cyst formation, occur due to increased mechanical stress on the underlying bone. Cartilage breakdown triggers the release of inflammatory mediators such as interleukin-1 (IL-1) and tumor necrosis factor-alpha (TNF-α), leading to synovial inflammation and joint tenderness. Increased vascularity in the synovium contributes to inflammation and discomfort, further perpetuating the condition [80, 116, 117].

Treatment Options

Management of metatarsal OA focuses on pain relief, improving mobility, and preventing further joint degeneration [86, 118–122]:

- *Non-Pharmacological*:
  - *Footwear Modifications*:
    Shoes with a wide toe box, cushioning, and stiff soles to reduce pressure on the metatarsal joints
    Rocker-bottom shoes to facilitate walking and reduce joint motion
  - *Orthotics*:
    Custom insoles or metatarsal pads to offload pressure from the affected joints
  - *Physical Therapy*:
    Stretching and strengthening exercises for foot and calf muscles
    Range-of-motion exercises to maintain joint mobility.
  - *Activity Modification*:
    Avoiding high-impact activities or prolonged standing
    Incorporating low-impact exercises like swimming or cycling
  - *Weight Management*:
    Reducing body weight to minimize stress on the forefoot
- *Pharmacological*:
  - NSAIDs for pain relief and inflammation control
  - Topical analgesics like capsaicin or diclofenac gel for localized symptom management
  - Corticosteroid injections for acute inflammation and severe pain
- *Procedural/Surgical*:
  - *Cheilectomy*:
    Removal of bone spurs and other impediments to improve joint motion, particularly in the first MTP joint
  - *Arthrodesis*:
    Joint fusion to relieve pain in advanced cases, though it limits motion
  - *Joint Replacement*:
    Prosthetic replacement of the first MTP joint for pain relief and restoration of function
  - *Osteotomy*:
    Realignment surgery to redistribute joint load and correct deformities

- *Emerging Therapies*:
  - Platelet-rich plasma (PRP) injections for cartilage repair
  - Stem cell therapy to promote regeneration of damaged joint tissues
  - Biologic agents targeting inflammatory pathways

In conclusion, metatarsal OA is a debilitating condition that significantly impacts forefoot function and mobility. Early recognition and intervention with lifestyle modifications, physical therapy, and footwear adjustments are crucial for managing symptoms and preserving joint function. For advanced cases, surgical and regenerative therapies offer promising solutions for pain relief and improved quality of life.

Dochu algorithm: metatarsal osteoarthritis	
External landmarks	Palpaple tendon of the extensor hallucis longus muscle, palpable dorsal pedal artery
Probe positioning	Transverse probe orientation over the extensor hallucis longus tendon at the level of the intermalleolar line (Fig. 3.37)
Target vessel	Dorsal pedal artery (Figs. 3.38 and 3.39)
Needle size	27G, length: 19 mm
Medication	Imipenem/Cilastatin (1 vial: 0.5 g/0.5 g) diluted with 10 cc of saline
Dosage	1.0–1.5 ml
Cuff position	NA

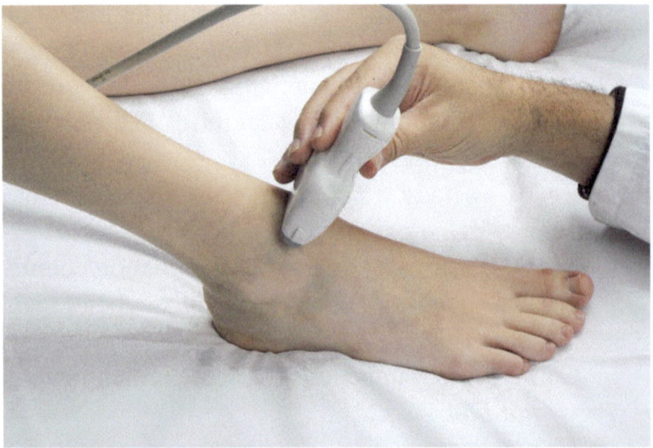

Fig. 3.37 Transverse probe orientation at the level of the intermalleolar line over the palpable dorsal pedal artery

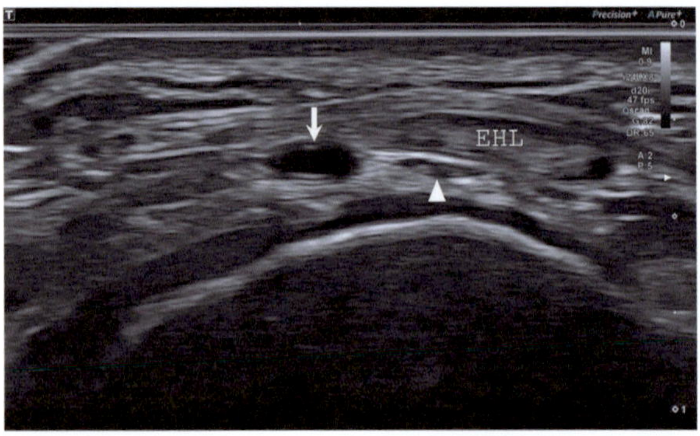

Fig. 3.38 Depiction of the dorsal pedal artery (arrow) lateral to the extensor hallucis longus tendon (EHL). Deep fibular nerve (arrowhead)

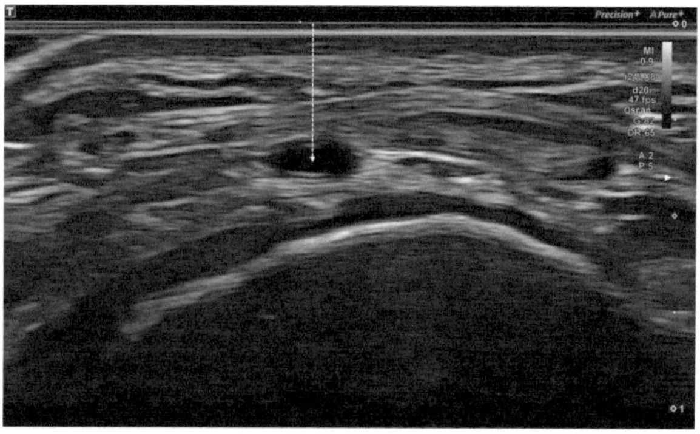

Fig. 3.39 Needle entry path in an out-of-plane access (dotted arrow)

Hallux Rigidus

Introduction

Hallux rigidus is a degenerative condition that affects the first metatarsophalangeal (MTP) joint at the base of the big toe. It is characterized by progressive stiffness, pain, and a loss of motion, primarily due to osteoarthritis. As the condition progresses, individuals may experience significant functional impairment, which can make activities involving toe movement, such as walking or running, increasingly difficult.

Epidemiology

Hallux rigidus is the most common arthritic condition affecting the big toe. It is associated with several risk factors. The prevalence of hallux rigidus is approximately 2.5% of the population, with higher rates observed in older adults. The condition typically occurs in individuals over the age of 30, and its prevalence increases with age. It is slightly more common in women. Risk factors for developing hallux rigidus include repetitive trauma or overuse, particularly among athletes or dancers. Structural foot abnormalities such as flat feet or high arches may also contribute, as can a genetic predisposition to osteoarthritis or joint disorders. A history of injuries, including fractures or sprains to the big toe, is another contributing factor.

Clinical Presentation and Symptoms

Hallux rigidus generally presents with symptoms that worsen over time. Pain is usually localized to the MTP joint, particularly during activities that involve dorsiflexion, such as walking or climbing stairs. In advanced stages, the pain may become constant, even during rest. Stiffness is also common, with limited range of motion, especially when attempting to bend the toe upward. This can make activities like running or squatting difficult. Swelling and tenderness around the MTP joint may be present, along with bony outgrowths (osteophytes) that can form at the joint, leading to visible deformities and further restricting motion. Patients may develop an altered gait, avoiding pushing off the big toe, which can result in compensatory walking patterns and cause pain in other areas of the foot or lower limbs. Functional limitations may also arise, such as difficulty wearing tight or heeled shoes due to pain or swelling.

Pathophysiology

Hallux rigidus arises from a combination of mechanical stress, joint degeneration, and inflammatory processes. Repeated stress or trauma to the MTP joint causes microdamage to the cartilage, leading to its degeneration. As the cartilage wears away, bone-on-bone contact occurs, which leads to pain and further joint erosion. Inflammation, mediated by cytokines, contributes to the breakdown of cartilage and joint swelling. In an attempt to stabilize the joint, the body forms bone spurs (osteophytes), which exacerbate stiffness and pain. Hypervascularity, or increased blood flow, occurs in the synovium as part of the inflammatory and reparative process, contributing to pain and swelling. Chronic degeneration leads to narrowing of the joint space and, in severe cases, ankylosis (fusion) of the joint.

Treatment Options

Management of hallux rigidus depends on the severity of symptoms and the extent of joint degeneration:

- *Non-Pharmacological*:
  - Use of footwear with a wide toe box and stiff soles to reduce pressure on the MTP joint
  - Custom orthotics to support the foot and offload pressure from the big toe
  - Physical therapy to stretch and strengthen the foot and lower limb muscles
  - Activity modification to avoid activities that exacerbate symptoms
- *Pharmacological*:
  - NSAIDs for pain relief and inflammation control
  - Topical analgesics, such as capsaicin cream, for localized pain management
  - Corticosteroid injections for temporary relief of inflammation and pain
- *Procedural/Surgical*:
  - Cheilectomy: Surgical removal of bone spurs to improve joint mobility and reduce pain

  - Arthrodesis: Joint fusion to eliminate pain in severe cases, though at the cost of motion
  - Joint Replacement: Prosthetic implants to restore joint function, typically for younger or more active patients
- *Emerging Therapies*:
  - Platelet-rich plasma (PRP) injections for cartilage repair
  - Stem cell therapy for regenerative healing
  - Biologic agents targeting inflammatory cytokines in cases with systemic inflammatory contributions

In conclusion, hallux rigidus is a debilitating condition that can severely impact mobility and quality of life. Early diagnosis and intervention with conservative treatments can often provide relief, while advanced surgical options and emerging regenerative therapies offer hope for improved outcomes in more severe cases.

Dochu algorithm: hallux rigidus	
External landmarks	Palpaple tendon of the extensor hallucis longus muscle, palpable dorsal pedal artery
Probe positioning	Transverse probe orientation over the extensor hallucis longus tendon at the level of the intermalleolar line (Fig. 3.40)
Target vessel	Dorsal pedal artery (Fig. 3.41 and 3.42)
Needle size	27G, length: 19 mm
Medication	Imipenem/Cilastatin (1vial: 0.5 g/0.5 g) diluted with 10 cc of saline
Dosage	1.0–1.5 ml
Cuff position	NA

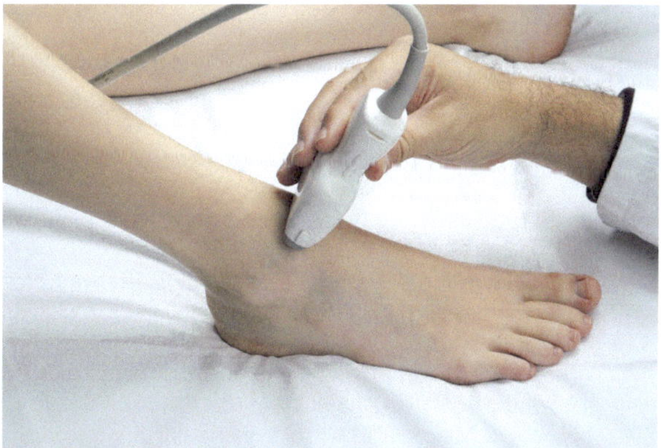

Fig. 3.40 Transverse probe orientation at the level of the intermalleolar line over the palpable dorsal pedal artery

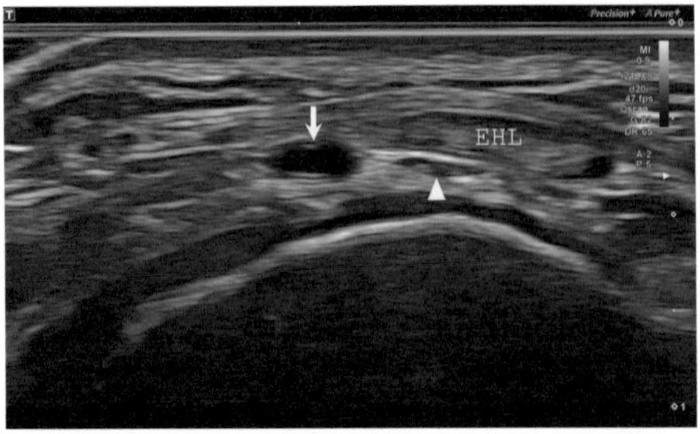

Fig. 3.41 Depiction of the dorsal pedal artery (arrow) lateral to the extensor hallucis longus tendon (EHL). Deep fibular nerve (arrowhead)

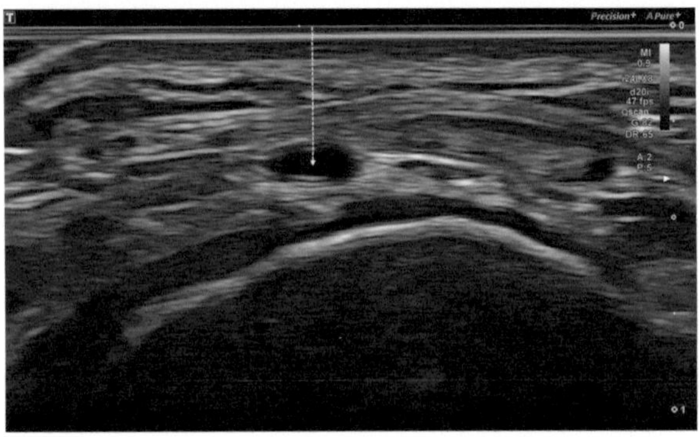

Fig. 3.42 Needle entry path in an out-of-plane access (dotted arrow)

References

1. Speers CJ, Bhogal GS. Greater trochanteric pain syndrome: a review of diagnosis and management in general practice. Br J Gen Pract. 2017;67(663):479–80.
2. Redmond JM, Chen AW, Domb BG. Greater trochanteric pain syndrome. J Am Acad Orthop Surg. 2016;24(4):231–40.
3. Strauss EJ, Nho SJ, Kelly BT. Greater trochanteric pain syndrome. Sports Med Arthrosc Rev. 2010;18(2):113–9.
4. Segal NA, Felson DT, Torner JC, Zhu Y, Curtis JR, Niu J, Nevitt MC, Group, M.O.M.S. Greater trochanteric pain syndrome: epidemiology and associated factors. Arch Phys Med Rehabil. 2007;88(8):988–92.
5. Williams BS, Cohen SP. Greater trochanteric pain syndrome: a review of anatomy, diagnosis and treatment. Anesth Analg. 2009;108(5):1662–70.
6. Shbeeb MI, Matteson EL. Trochanteric bursitis (greater trochanter pain syndrome). Mayo Clin Proc. 1996;71(6):565–9. Elsevier.
7. Schapira D, Nahir M, Scharf Y. Trochanteric bursitis: a common clinical problem. Arch Phys Med Rehabil. 1986;67(11):815–7.
8. Guemara R, Nissen MJ. The greater trochanteric pain syndrome: clinical presentation, diagnosis, and management. Curr Treat Options Rheumatol. 2023;9(4):192–203.
9. Gomez LP, Li DD, Childress JM. Greater trochanteric pain syndrome (greater trochanteric bursitis). In: StatPearls [internet]. StatPearls Publishing; 2024.

10. Aaron DL, Patel A, Kayiaros S, Calfee R. Four common types of bursitis: diagnosis and management. J Am Acad Orthop Surg. 2011;19(6):359–67.
11. Ho GWK, Howard TM. Greater trochanteric pain syndrome: more than bursitis and iliotibial tract friction. Curr Sports Med Rep. 2012;11(5):232–8.
12. Geneen LJ, Moore RA, Clarke C, Martin D, Colvin LA, Smith BH. Physical activity and exercise for chronic pain in adults: an overview of Cochrane reviews. Cochrane Database Syst Rev. 2017;4(4):CD011279.
13. Lustenberger DP, Ng VY, Best TM, Ellis TJ. Efficacy of treatment of trochanteric bursitis: a systematic review. Clin J Sport Med. 2011;21(5):447–53.
14. Rasmussen KJE, Fanø N. Trochanteric bursitis: treatment by corticosteroid injection. Scand J Rheumatol. 1985;14(4):417–20.
15. Heidari B. Knee osteoarthritis prevalence, risk factors, pathogenesis and features: part I. Caspian J Intern Med. 2011;2(2):205.
16. Losina E, Weinstein AM, Reichmann WM, Burbine SA, Solomon DH, Daigle ME, Rome BN, Chen SP, Hunter DJ, Suter LG, Jordan JM. Lifetime risk and age at diagnosis of symptomatic knee osteoarthritis in the US. Arthritis Care Res. 2013;65(5):703–11.
17. Zhang Y, Jordan JM. Epidemiology of osteoarthritis. Clin Geriatr Med. 2010;26(3):355–69.
18. Neogi T. The epidemiology and impact of pain in osteoarthritis. Osteoarthr Cartil. 2013;21(9):1145–53.
19. Thirumaran AJ, Deveza LA, Atukorala I, Hunter DJ. Assessment of pain in osteoarthritis of the knee. J Pers Med. 2023;13(7):1139.
20. Gerena LA, Mabrouk A, DeCastro A. Knee effusion. In: StatPearls [internet]. StatPearls Publishing; 2024.
21. Lee PYF, Nixion A, Chandratreya A, Murray JM. Synovial plica syndrome of the knee: a commonly overlooked cause of anterior knee pain. The Surgery Journal. 2017;3(01):e9–e16.
22. Vincent KR, Conrad BP, Fregly BJ, Vincent HK. The pathophysiology of osteoarthritis: a mechanical perspective on the knee joint. PM&R. 2012;4(5):S3–9.
23. Zeng CY, Zhang ZR, Tang ZM, Hua FZ. Benefits and mechanisms of exercise training for knee osteoarthritis. Front Physiol. 2021;12:794062.
24. Mora JC, Przkora R, Cruz-Almeida Y. Knee osteoarthritis: pathophysiology and current treatment modalities. J Pain Res. 2018;11:2189–96.
25. Ringdahl E, Pandit S. Treatment of knee osteoarthritis. Am Fam Physician. 2011;83(11):1287–92.
26. Katz JN, Arant KR, Loeser RF. Diagnosis and treatment of hip and knee osteoarthritis: a review. JAMA. 2021;325(6):568–78.
27. Kan HS, Chan PK, Chiu KY, Yan CH, Yeung SS, Ng YL, Shiu KW, Ho T. Non-surgical treatment of knee osteoarthritis. Hong Kong Med J. 2019;25:127.
28. Zaia B, Gharahbaghian L. Patellar tendonitis. West J Emerg Med. 2011;12(1):139.
29. Zwerver J, Bredeweg SW, Van Den Akker-Scheek I. Prevalence of Jumper's knee among nonelite athletes from different sports: a cross-sectional survey. Am J Sports Med. 2011;39(9):1984–8.
30. Walton J, Kozina E, Woo F, Jadidi S. A review of patellar tendinopathy in athletes involved in jumping sports. Cureus. 2023;15(10):e47459.
31. Malliaras P, Cook J, Purdam C, Rio E. Patellar tendinopathy: clinical diagnosis, load management, and advice for challenging case presentations. J Orthop Sports Phys Ther. 2015;45(11):887–98.
32. Lian ØB, Engebretsen L, Bahr R. Prevalence of jumper's knee among elite athletes from different sports: a cross-sectional study. Am J Sports Med. 2005;33(4):561–7.
33. Antich TJ, Randall CC, Westbrook RA, Morrissey MC, Brewster CE. Evaluation of knee extensor mechanism disorders: clinical presentation of 112 patients. J Orthop Sports Phys Ther. 1986;8(5):248–54.

34. Pierets K, Verdonk R, De Muynck M, Lagast J. Jumper's knee: postoperative assessment a retrospective clinical study: a retrospective clinical study. Knee Surg Sports Traumatol Arthrosc. 1999;7:239–42.
35. Fredberg U, Bolvig L. Jumper's knee: review of the literature. Scand J Med Sci Sports. 1999;9(2):66–73.
36. Rosso F, Bonasia DE, Cottino U, Dettoni F, Bruzzone M, Rossi R. Patellar tendon: from tendinopathy to rupture. Asia-Pacific J Sports Med Arthrosc Rehabil Technol. 2015;2(4):99–107.
37. Fredberg U, Stengaard-Pedersen K. Chronic tendinopathy tissue pathology, pain mechanisms, and etiology with a special focus on inflammation. Scand J Med Sci Sports. 2008;18(1):3–15.
38. Abate M, Gravare Silbernagel K, Siljeholm C, Di Iorio A, De Amicis D, Salini V, Werner S, Paganelli R. Pathogenesis of tendinopathies: inflammation or degeneration? Arthritis Res Ther. 2009;11:1–15.
39. Muaidi QI. Rehabilitation of patellar tendinopathy. J Musculoskelet Neuronal Interact. 2020;20(4):535.
40. Rosen AB, Wellsandt E, Nicola M, Tao MA. Clinical management of patellar tendinopathy. J Athl Train. 2022;57(7):621–31.
41. Rodriguez-Merchan EC. The treatment of patellar tendinopathy. J Orthop Traumatol. 2013;14:77–81.
42. Figueroa D, Figueroa F, Calvo R. Patellar tendinopathy: diagnosis and treatment. J Am Acad Orthop Surg. 2016;24(12):e184–92.
43. Everhart JS, Cole D, Sojka JH, Higgins JD, Magnussen RA, Schmitt LC, Flanigan DC. Treatment options for patellar tendinopathy: a systematic review. Arthroscopy. 2017;33(4):861–72.
44. Mohseni M, Mabrouk A, Li DD, Graham C. Pes anserine bursitis. In: StatPearls [internet]. StatPearls Publishing; 2024.
45. Alvarez-Nemegyei J. Risk factors for pes anserinus tendinitis/bursitis syndrome: a case control study. JCR J Clin Rheumatol. 2007;13(2):63–5.
46. Rennie WJ, Saifuddin A. Pes anserine bursitis: incidence in symptomatic knees and clinical presentation. Skeletal Radiol. 2005;34:395–8.
47. Sarifakioglu B, Afsar SI, Yalbuzdag SA, Ustaömer K, Bayramoğlu M. Comparison of the efficacy of physical therapy and corticosteroid injection in the treatment of pes anserine tendino-bursitis. J Phys Ther Sci. 2016;28(7):1993–7.
48. Saggini R, Di Stefano A, Dodaj I, Scarcello L, Bellomo RG. Pes anserine bursitis in symptomatic osteoarthritis patients: a mesotherapy treatment study. J Altern Complement Med. 2015;21(8):480–4.
49. Lee JH, Kim KJ, Jeong YG, Lee NS, Han SY, Lee CG, Kim KY, Han SH. Pes anserinus and anserine bursa: anatomical study. Anat Cell Biol. 2014;47(2):127–31.
50. Hunter CW, Deer TR, Jones MR, Chang Chien GC, D'Souza RS, Davis T, Eldon ER, Esposito MF, Goree JH, Hewan-Lowe L, Maloney JA. Consensus guidelines on interventional therapies for knee pain (STEP guidelines) from the American Society of Pain and Neuroscience. J Pain Res. 2022:2683–745.
51. Fredericson M, Wolf C. Iliotibial band syndrome in runners: innovations in treatment. Sports Med. 2005;35:451–9.
52. Strauss EJ, Kim S, Calcei JG, Park D. Iliotibial band syndrome: evaluation and management. J Am Acad Orthop Surg. 2011;19(12):728–36.
53. Hutchinson LA, Lichtwark GA, Willy RW, Kelly LA. The iliotibial band: a complex structure with versatile functions. Sports Med. 2022;52(5):995–1008.
54. Van der Worp MP, van der Horst N, de Wijer A, Backx FJ, Nijhuis-van der Sanden MW. Iliotibial band syndrome in runners: a systematic review. Sports Med. 2012;42:969–92.
55. Lavine R. Iliotibial band friction syndrome. Curr Rev Musculoskelet Med. 2010;3(1):18–22.

56. Holmes JC, Pruitt AL, Whalen NJ. Iliotibial band syndrome in cyclists. Am J Sports Med. 1993;21(3):419–24.
57. Beals C, Flanigan D. A review of treatments for iliotibial band syndrome in the athletic population. Journal of sports medicine. 2013;2013(1):367169.
58. Baker RL, Souza RB, Fredericson M. Iliotibial band syndrome: soft tissue and biomechanical factors in evaluation and treatment. PM&R. 2011;3(6):550–61.
59. Friede MC, Innerhofer G, Fink C, Alegre LM, Csapo R. Conservative treatment of iliotibial band syndrome in runners: are we targeting the right goals? Phys Ther Sport. 2022;54:44–52.
60. Fredericson M, Guillet M, DeBenedictis L. Quick solutions for iliotibial band syndrome. Phys Sportsmed. 2000;28(2):52–68.
61. Sanchez-Alvarado A, Bokil C, Cassel M, Engel T. Effects of conservative treatment strategies for iliotibial band syndrome on pain and function in runners: a systematic review. Front Sports Act Living. 2024;6:1386456.
62. Melanson SW, Shuman VL. Acute ankle sprain. In: StatPearls [internet]. StatPearls Publishing; 2023.
63. Herzog MM, Kerr ZY, Marshall SW, Wikstrom EA. Epidemiology of ankle sprains and chronic ankle instability. J Athl Train. 2019;54(6):603–10.
64. Jungmann PM, Lange T, Wenning M, Baumann FA, Bamberg F, Jung M. Ankle sprains in athletes: current epidemiological, clinical and imaging trends. Open Access J Sports Med. 2023;14:29–46.
65. Fong DTP, Man CY, Yung PSH, Cheung SY, Chan KM. Sport-related ankle injuries attending an accident and emergency department. Injury. 2008;39(10):1222–7.
66. Polzer H, Kanz KG, Prall WC, Haasters F, Ockert B, Mutschler W, Grote S. Diagnosis and treatment of acute ankle injuries: development of an evidence-based algorithm. Orthop Rev. 2011;4(1):e5.
67. Michels F, Wastyn H, Pottel H, Stockmans F, Vereecke E, Matricali G. The presence of persistent symptoms 12 months following a first lateral ankle sprain: a systematic review and meta-analysis. Foot Ankle Surg. 2022;28(7):817–26.
68. Hubbard TJ, Wikstrom EA. Ankle sprain: pathophysiology, predisposing factors, and management strategies. Open Access J Sports Med. 2010;1:115–22.
69. Fong DT, Chan YY, Mok KM, Yung PS, Chan KM. Understanding acute ankle ligamentous sprain injury in sports. BMC Sports Sci Med Rehabil. 2009;1:1–14.
70. Ortega-Avila AB, Cervera-Garvi P, Marchena-Rodrıguez A, Chicharro-Luna E, Nester CJ, Starbuck C, Gijon-Nogueron G. Conservative treatment for acute ankle sprain: a systematic review. J Clin Med. 2020;9(10):3128.
71. Doherty C, Bleakley C, Delahunt E, Holden S. Treatment and prevention of acute and recurrent ankle sprain: an overview of systematic reviews with meta-analysis. Br J Sports Med. 2017;51(2):113–25.
72. Kemler E, van de Port I, Backx F, van Dijk CN. A systematic review on the treatment of acute ankle sprain: brace versus other functional treatment types. Sports Med. 2011;41:185–97.
73. Soboroff, S.H., Pappius, E.M. And Komaroff, A.L., 1984. Benefits, risks, and costs of alternative approaches to the evaluation and treatment of severe ankle sprain. Clin Orthop Relat Res, 183, pp.160–168.
74. Herrera-Pérez M, Valderrabano V, Godoy-Santos AL, de César Netto C, González-Martín D, Tejero S. Ankle osteoarthritis: comprehensive review and treatment algorithm proposal. EFORT Open Rev. 2022;7(7):448–59.
75. Herrera-Pérez M, González-Martín D, Vallejo-Márquez M, Godoy-Santos AL, Valderrabano V, Tejero S. Ankle osteoarthritis aetiology. J Clin Med. 2021;10(19):4489.
76. Kiely PD, Lloyd ME. Ankle arthritis–an important signpost in rheumatologic practice. Rheumatology. 2021;60(1):23–33.
77. Hunter DJ, McDougall JJ, Keefe FJ. The symptoms of osteoarthritis and the genesis of pain. Rheum Dis Clin North Am. 2008;34(3):623–43.

78. Mugno AT, Constant D. Recurrent ankle sprain. In: StatPearls [internet]. StatPearls Publishing; 2020.
79. Le V, Veljkovic A, Salat P, Wing K, Penner M, Younger A. Ankle arthritis. Foot Ankle Orthop. 2019;4(3):2473011419852931.
80. Buckwalter JA, Anderson DD, Brown TD, Tochigi Y, Martin JA. The roles of mechanical stresses in the pathogenesis of osteoarthritis: implications for treatment of joint injuries. Cartilage. 2013;4(4):286–94.
81. Delco ML, Kennedy JG, Bonassar LJ, Fortier LA. Post-traumatic osteoarthritis of the ankle: a distinct clinical entity requiring new research approaches. J Orthop Res. 2017;35(3):440–53.
82. Miller RE, Miller RJ, Malfait AM. Osteoarthritis joint pain: the cytokine connection. Cytokine. 2014;70(2):185–93.
83. Chow YY, Chin KY. The role of inflammation in the pathogenesis of osteoarthritis. Mediat Inflamm. 2020;2020(1):8293921.
84. Tejero S, Prada-Chamorro E, González-Martín D, García-Guirao A, Galhoum A, Valderrabano V, Herrera-Pérez M. Conservative treatment of ankle osteoarthritis. J Clin Med. 2021;10(19):4561.
85. Schmid T, Krause FG. Conservative treatment of asymmetric ankle osteoarthritis. Foot Ankle Clin. 2013;18(3):437–48.
86. Paterson KL, Gates L. Clinical assessment and management of foot and ankle osteoarthritis: a review of current evidence and focus on pharmacological treatment. Drugs Aging. 2019;36:203–11.
87. Godoy-Santos AL, Fonseca LF, Cesar CD, Giordano V, Valderrabano V, Rammelt S. Ankle osteoarthritis. Rev Bras Ortop. 2021;56(06):689–96.
88. Weaver JS, Vina ER, Munk PL, Klauser AS, Elifritz JM, Taljanovic MS. Gouty arthropathy: review of clinical manifestations and treatment, with emphasis on imaging. J Clin Med. 2021;11(1):166.
89. Ragab G, Elshahaly M, Bardin T. Gout: an old disease in new perspective–a review. J Adv Res. 2017;8(5):495–511.
90. Asghari KM, Zahmatyar M, Seyedi F, Motamedi A, Zolfi M, Alamdary SJ, Fazlollahi A, Shamekh A, Mousavi SE, Nejadghaderi SA, Mohammadinasab R. Gout: global epidemiology, risk factors, comorbidities and complications: a narrative review. BMC Musculoskelet Disord. 2024;25:1047.
91. Doherty M. New insights into the epidemiology of gout. Rheumatology. 2009;48(suppl_2):ii2–8.
92. Hospital for Special Surgery (HSS), 2024. Gout: risk factors, diagnosis, and treatment. [online] Available at: https://www.hss.edu/conditions_gout-risk-factors-diagnosis-treatment.asp [Accessed 29 December 2024].
93. Wortmann RL. Gout and hyperuricemia. Curr Opin Rheumatol. 2002;14(3):281–6.
94. Ahn EY, So MW. The pathogenesis of gout. J Rheum Dis. 2024;32(1):8.
95. Coburn BW, Mikuls TR. Treatment options for acute gout. Fed Pract. 2016;33(1):35.
96. Schlesinger N, Dalbeth N, Perez-Ruiz F. Gout–what are the treatment options? Expert Opin Pharmacother. 2009;10(8):1319–28.
97. Schlesinger N. The safety of treatment options available for gout. Expert Opin Drug Saf. 2017;16(4):429–36.
98. Pillinger MH, Mandell BF. Therapeutic approaches in the treatment of gout. Semin Arthritis Rheum. 2020;50(3):S24–30. WB Saunders.
99. Cronstein BN, Terkeltaub R. The inflammatory process of gout and its treatment. Arthritis Res Ther. 2006;8:1–7.
100. DeMaio M, Paine R, Drez DJ. Achilles tendonitis. Orthopedics. 1995;18(2):195–204.
101. Malliaras P. Physiotherapy management of Achilles tendinopathy. J Physiother. 2022;68(4):221–37.
102. Schwartz EN, Su J. Plantar fasciitis: a concise review. Perm J. 2014;18(1):e105.
103. Trojian T, Tucker AK. Plantar fasciitis. Am Fam Physician. 2019;99(12):744–50.

104. Littlejohn B. From heel to toe: investigating plantar fasciitis causes, diagnosis, and treatment strategies. 2024.
105. Latt LD, Jaffe DE, Tang Y, Taljanovic MS. Evaluation and treatment of chronic plantar fasciitis. Foot Ankle Orthop. 2020;5(1):2473011419896763.
106. Tseng WC, Chen YC, Lee TM, Chen WS. Plantar fasciitis: an updated review. J Med Ultrasound. 2023;31(4):268–74.
107. Lim AT, How CH, Tan B. Management of plantar fasciitis in the outpatient setting. Singapore Med J. 2016;57(4):168.
108. Rathleff MS, Mølgaard CM, Fredberg U, Kaalund S, Andersen KB, Jensen TT, Aaskov S, Olesen JL. High-load strength training improves outcome in patients with plantar fasciitis: a randomized controlled trial with 12-month follow-up. Scand J Med Sci Sports. 2015;25(3):e292–300.
109. Koc TA Jr, Bise CG, Neville C, Carreira D, Martin RL, McDonough CM. Heel pain–plantar fasciitis: revision 2023: clinical practice guidelines linked to the international classification of functioning, disability and health from the academy of orthopaedic physical therapy and American academy of sports physical therapy of the American physical therapy association. J Orthop Sports Phys Ther. 2023;53(12):CPG1 CPG39.
110. Allan JJ, McClelland JA, Munteanu SE, Buldt AK, Landorf KB, Roddy E, Auhl M, Menz HB. First metatarsophalangeal joint range of motion is associated with lower limb kinematics in individuals with first metatarsophalangeal joint osteoarthritis. J Foot Ankle Res. 2020;13:1–8.
111. Kalichman L, Hernández-Molina G. Midfoot and forefoot osteoarthritis. Foot. 2014;24(3):128–34.
112. Senga Y, Nishimura A, Ito N, Kitaura Y, Sudo A. Prevalence of and risk factors for hallux rigidus: a cross-sectional study in Japan. BMC Musculoskelet Disord. 2021;22:1–7.
113. Foot I, Arnold JB, Bowen CJ, Chapman LS, Gates LS, Golightly YM, Halstead J, Hannan MT, Menz HB, Munteanu SE, Paterson KL. International Foot and Ankle Osteoarthritis Consortium review and research agenda for diagnosis, epidemiology, burden, outcome assessment and treatment. Osteoarthr Cartil. 2022;30(7):945–55.
114. Lee KT, Park YU, Jegal H, Young KW, Kim JS, Lim SY. Osteoarthritis of the second metatarsophalangeal joint associated with hallux valgus deformity. Foot Ankle Int. 2014;35(12):1329–33.
115. Bergin SM, Munteanu SE, Zammit GV, Nikolopoulos N, Menz HB. Impact of first metatarsophalangeal joint osteoarthritis on health-related quality of life. Arthritis Care Res. 2012;64(11):1691–8.
116. He Y, Li Z, Alexander PG, Ocasio-Nieves BD, Yocum L, Lin H, Tuan RS. Pathogenesis of osteoarthritis: risk factors, regulatory pathways in chondrocytes, and experimental models. Biology. 2020;9(8):194.
117. Li G, Yin J, Gao J, Cheng TS, Pavlos NJ, Zhang C, Zheng MH. Subchondral bone in osteoarthritis: insight into risk factors and microstructural changes. Arthritis Res Ther. 2013;15:1–12.
118. Menz HB, Auhl M, Tan JM, Levinger P, Roddy E, Munteanu SE. Effectiveness of foot orthoses versus rocker-sole footwear for first metatarsophalangeal joint osteoarthritis: randomized trial. Arthritis Care Res. 2016;68(5):581–9.
119. Frecklington M, Dalbeth N, McNair P, Gow P, Williams A, Carroll M, Rome K. Footwear interventions for foot pain, function, impairment and disability for people with foot and ankle arthritis: a literature review. Semin Arthritis Rheum. 2018;47(6):814–24. WB Saunders.
120. Jung HG, Myerson MS, Schon LC. Spectrum of operative treatments and clinical outcomes for atraumatic osteoarthritis of the tarsometatarsal joints. Foot Ankle Int. 2007;28(4):482–9.
121. Jung HG, Jeon SH, Kim TH, Park JT. Total ankle arthroplasty with combined calcaneal and metatarsal osteotomies for treatment of ankle osteoarthritis with accompanying cavovarus deformities: early results. Foot Ankle Int. 2013;34(1):140–7.

122. Deschamps K, Mercken K, Verschuren P, Eerdekens M, Vanstraelen E, Wuite S, Matricali GA. Foot biomechanics in patients with advanced subtalar-and mid-tarsal joint osteoarthritis and poorly responding to conservative treatment. J Foot Ankle Res. 2023;16(1):85.

MIX
Papier aus verantwortungsvollen Quellen
Paper from responsible sources
FSC® C105338

If you have any concerns about our products,
you can contact us on
ProductSafety@springernature.com

In case Publisher is established outside the EU,
the EU authorized representative is:
Springer Nature Customer Service Center GmbH
Europaplatz 3, 69115 Heidelberg, Germany

Printed by Libri Plureos GmbH
in Hamburg, Germany